Praise for *Mindfulness-Based Stress Reduction*

"We can feel the decades of experience inside the MBSR classroom that Lehrhaupt and Meibert call upon as they share the challenges and joys of engaging deeply with our lives that mindfulness affords us. They offer us a book of remarkable clarity and precision about a topic that's difficult to express. It's a powerful reminder of the importance and centrality of turning toward our life experience with nonjudgmental awareness, insight, and curiosity supported by wise teachers and a safe space. It's a great thing when those teachers can reach us from the pages of a book and encourage us onward. As it always is, the time for mindfulness is now!"

— Tim Burnett, founder and executive director of Mindfulness Northwest

"There are many books on mindfulness — but this one uniquely offers a clear, session-by-session layout of the MBSR curriculum. The text is brought to life by the examples of the participants' experiences with the process and the authors' experiences as teachers. The book will be invaluable to people taking the MBSR course, as well as to MBSR trainees and seasoned teachers alike."

— Rebecca Crane, PhD, director of the
Centre for Mindfulness Research & Practice, Bangor, Wales

"This valuable and no-nonsense book will definitely be of great value to everyone exploring mindfulness, whether they are curious beginners, participants of mindfulness courses, or regular practitioners. The wise and straightforward explanations of what this is all about will assist the reader in discovering the basic truths of the practice and the in-depth mysteries that lie at the heart of pure presence. Two experienced and wise teachers are offering their service, and we should all be grateful for their effort in making this guidebook available to us all."

— Michael de Vibe, MD, PhD, cofounder of Mindfulness Norway

"Arguably the most concise and revealing description of MBSR to date, this book is the precious fruit of the authors' decades of experience teaching MBSR. Readers will learn the rationale and key practices of each session, see how the sessions are elegantly woven together, find answers to common misconceptions, and discover ways to overcome obstacles to prac way into all aspects of modern society, this book nating insight into what started it all."

— Christopher Germer, PhD, cofou
Self-Compassion, founding membe
and Psychotherapy, and author of *The Mindful Path to Self-Compassion*

"A powerful and accessible book on mindfulness that will serve all."
— Rev. Joan Halifax, abbot of Upaya Zen Center

"This book does a magnificent job of rendering not only the curriculum of MBSR but, even more importantly, its *feeling tone*, gently emphasizing that it takes energy and sustained commitment to practice and embody mindfulness. I am grateful that this book is now available as a skillful gateway into MBSR, mindfulness, and one's own life in the face of stress, pain, illness, and the human condition itself."
— Jon Kabat-Zinn, founder of MBSR and author of
Full Catastrophe Living and *Coming to Our Senses*

"This is a comprehensive and highly readable resource for all those who are contemplating an eight-week MBSR program as well as for anybody who is familiar with the adventure of an MBSR course, teachers and participants alike. I will happily recommend this book to our teacher trainees and participants. It not only guides us in a thorough overview of the journey of MBSR but also shares with us a rich week-by-week description of the process, participants' experiences, and the deep wisdom of two skilled and highly immersed mindfulness teachers."
— Linda Kantor, director of the
Institute for Mindfulness South Africa (IMISA)

"This is a unique practice book, one to return to again and again. It reveals a series of very practical, powerful practices that anyone can incorporate into their daily life. As pointed out in the book, people who practice them regularly can more easily cope with the stress, strains, and struggles of modern life. For people contemplating taking an MBSR course, this book offers a great introduction and sense of what the experience might be like. For those taking an MBSR course, it will help enormously for exploring the themes presented in the classes. *Mindfulness-Based Stress Reduction* is a very important addition to the literature for the course."
— Sr. Stanislaus Kennedy, founder of The Sanctuary, Dublin, and author of
Day by Day, *Seasons of Hope*, and *The Road Home*

"Linda Lehrhaupt and Petra Meibert have given us a beautifully articulated description of the mindfulness-based stress reduction approach enriched with anecdotes and quotes that bring it vividly to life — just as the practice of mindfulness can bring each of us fully to life. This book is an accessible and engaging invitation to explore the mindful relief of suffering and stress in a way that also offers the possibility of freedom, contentment, and peace."

— Maura Kenny, PhD, Mindfulness Training Institute Australasia

"In this book, two very experienced practitioners and senior teachers skillfully explain the essence of the renowned mindfulness-based stress reduction program. The result is a wonderful introduction and invitation for those who seek inner ease and freedom from stress and (chronic) pain. The strength of this heartwarming book lies in its simplicity and compassionate clarity. I recommend reading this jewel to anybody who wishes to start and explore this journey."

— Frits Koster, Vipassana meditation teacher, trainer of MBSR and MBCT, codeveloper of the Mindfulness-Based Compassionate Living program, author of *Liberating Insight* and *Buddhist Meditation in Stress Management*, and coauthor of *Mindfulness-Based Compassionate Living*

"This well-structured, helpful, and practical book takes readers through the eight-week MBSR course, providing detailed descriptions of the practices and inspiring examples of students' experiences. The authors have distilled their decades of teaching experience and deep understanding of MBSR into simple, intimate, friendly, and accessible language. The book is an embodiment of mindfulness itself."

— S. Helen Ma, PhD, founding teacher of Hong Kong Center for Mindfulness

"In their book, Linda Lehrhaupt and Petra Meibert provide a clear compass for anyone interested in enhancing health and wellness by engaging with the practices and principles of MBSR. For those who have already attended and completed the MBSR program, this book can serve to renew, refresh, and reinforce earlier learning. Ultimately, it is a guide for all who choose to live with greater awareness and compassion."

— Florence Meleo-Meyer, MS, MA, coauthor of *A Mindfulness-Based Stress Reduction Workbook for Anxiety* and *The MBSR Home Study Course* and director of the Train-the-Trainer Program at Oasis Institute for Mindfulness-Based Professional Education and Training at the Center for Mindfulness in Medicine, Health Care, and Society, University of Massachusetts Medical School

"As a meditation teacher with over forty-five years of experience, primarily in traditional Japanese Zen, I've found this work to be incredibly clear and useful for those wishing to learn more about and practice MBSR. As mindfulness is the foundation of all systems of meditation, this will be a wonderful resource for teachers from all traditions. Congratulations to Linda Lehrhaupt and Petra Meibert for creating this concise guide!"

— Sensei Al Fusho Rapaport, Open Mind Zen Meditation Center,
Melbourne, FL

"This wonderful book is very accessible for those interested in mindfulness and MBSR as well as for MBSR teachers in training and trained teachers. Its detailed description of the MBSR curriculum and specific examples are supportive and practical. This book reflects the compassionate tone of MBSR in a beautiful way. It is a gift for all those who are interested in MBSR and who are on an inner journey to deal more skillfully and be more at ease with stress, pain, and illness. May it be of great benefit to all."

— Johan Tinge, director of the Instituut voor Mindfulness, the Netherlands

"This is a book about how to be in touch, moment by moment, with the actuality of your life, and to do so in a way that is kind to both yourself and others. Based on the hugely influential program of Jon Kabat-Zinn, the book wonderfully captures the essence of the mindfulness approach and promises to excite the interest of a new generation. Both authors are highly respected teachers and teacher trainers in mindfulness. Written in a beautifully accessible style, it will become a vital companion to those who follow its wise guidance. I highly recommend it to you."

— Mark Williams, emeritus professor of clinical psychology
at the University of Oxford and coauthor of
The Mindful Way through Depression

"What a great addition to the 'mindfulness shelf'! Linda Lehrhaupt and Petra Meibert take you gently by the hand and lead you through the classic eight-week MBSR curriculum. Sprinkled throughout the book are moving testimonies by course participants of how these practices changed their lives. These, plus the authors' personal and professional vignettes, clarify the concepts presented and attest to the power of the approach. Whether you are currently taking the course or you want to reinforce and deepen prior learning, this book is like having your own MBSR teacher standing beside you on your journey to enhanced health and well-being."

— Dina Wyshogrod, PhD, founder/director of MBSR-ISRAEL,
The Israeli Center for Mindfulness-Based Stress Reduction

Mindfulness-Based Stress Reduction

Mindfulness-Based Stress Reduction

The MBSR Program for Enhancing
Health and Vitality

LINDA LEHRHAUPT, PhD
PETRA MEIBERT, Dipl. Psych.

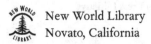
New World Library
Novato, California

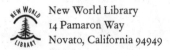
New World Library
14 Pamaron Way
Novato, California 94949

The material in this book is intended for education. It is not meant to take the place of diagnosis and treatment by a qualified medical practitioner or therapist. No expressed or implied guarantee of the effects of the use of the recommendations can be given or liability taken. The authors recommend that you consult with your doctor or other health-care provider to confirm that the MBSR program and, particularly, yoga are suitable for you. The authors are not liable for the results of consulting any of the individuals, organizations, or websites listed in this book. The listings are presented as a service but are not meant to be endorsements by the authors.

This book was originally published in German under the title *Stress bewältigen mit Achtsamkeit: Zu innerer Ruhe kommen durch MBSR* (Kösel Publications, 2010). It has been updated and new sections have been added.

Text design by Tona Pearce Myers

Library of Congress Cataloging-in-Publication Data
Names: Lehrhaupt, Linda Myoki, author. | Meibert, Petra.
Title: Mindfulness-based stress reduction : the MBSR program for enhancing health and
   vitality / Linda Lehrhaupt, PhD., Petra Meibert, Dipl. Psych.
Description: Novato, California : New World Library, [2017] | Includes index.
Identifiers: LCCN 2016052813 (print) | LCCN 2016053670 (ebook) | ISBN
   9781608684793 (paperback) | ISBN 9781608684809 (Ebook)
Subjects: LCSH: Stress management. | Mind and body. | Alternative medicine. |
  BISAC: SELF-HELP / Stress Management. | BODY, MIND & SPIRIT / Meditation.
  | HEALTH & FITNESS / Healthy Living. | HEALTH & FITNESS / Alternative
  Therapies.
Classification: LCC RA785 .L45 2017 (print) | LCC RA785 (ebook) | DDC
  155.9/042—dc23
LC record available at https://lccn.loc.gov/2016052813

First printing, March 2017
ISBN 978-1-60868-479-3
Ebook ISBN 978-1-60868-480-9
Printed in Canada on 100% postconsumer-waste recycled paper

New World Library is proud to be a Gold Certified Environmentally Responsible Publisher. Publisher certification awarded by Green Press Initiative.
www.greenpressinitiative.org

10   9   8   7   6   5   4   3   2

For Norbert and Taya.
Thank you for your trust and support. And for the laughter.

— L. L.

For Jörg.
Thank you for each day we share and for your honesty and friendship.

— P. M.

Contents

Introduction

If you have opened this book, then you may be experiencing what has become so widespread in our day and age: stress! Perhaps you feel overwhelmed and hope that Mindfulness-Based Stress Reduction will show you how to avoid what seems like an emotional avalanche. Perhaps you move through your day as if you are constantly in fifth gear without being able to stop or even downshift. Maybe it's exactly the opposite — something has caused you to pull the emergency brake, and your life has screeched to a halt. It could be the diagnosis of a serious illness, or losing your job or your home. It could also be relationship problems, a difficult work situation, or the strain of caring for a loved one.

Situations like these are among the many reasons why people enroll in a Mindfulness-Based Stress Reduction (MBSR) course. They are all circumstances in which we experience stress from events that catch us unaware and disrupt our lives, so that nothing is as it was before. Driven by a sense of urgency, we may search for solutions or become overwhelmed and give up on making any effort at all, sinking into complacency or paralysis. Our health may be affected: our blood pressure may rise, we may drink too much alcohol, overeat, or experience unexplained pain.

Many people who sign up for an MBSR course say they reached a point where they couldn't go on the way they had before. They felt a need to stop and shift direction. Others say they have lost touch with themselves and long for reconnection. They might be uncertain about what to do or how to do it, but one thing is clear: life can't continue the way it has.

In an MBSR course, participants are invited to connect deeply to their own lives. Practicing mindfulness means being present, awake, and aware. It means being in touch with the moment-to-moment stream of life in a nonjudgmental way that reflects kindness to ourselves and to the world at large. Rather than allow us to avoid or deny a difficult situation, mindfulness supports us so that we can be present in a situation as it unfolds.

This book is an introduction to MBSR. It presents both background information and some exercises. Our goals are to:

- explain the main elements of the eight-week MBSR course, which usually meets for two and a half to three hours once a week.
- provide instructions for practicing some of the exercises in an MBSR course.
- describe some of the basic theories about stress and demonstrate how mindfulness can help us be more balanced and centered in our lives.
- introduce mindfulness as a way of life.

Can you learn MBSR from a book? The answer is yes...and no. Practicing mindfulness — the core of MBSR — on your own is possible, and indeed many people have begun training by reading books, but a book is not a substitute for attending an MBSR class. There is tremendous value in practicing in a group and receiving guidance from a qualified teacher. A class can provide inspiration, motivation, and a more comprehensive view through interaction with others. An MBSR teacher and the group can help you explore your experience of the exercises and take you to a deeper level of understanding. Although a book may be a great starting point, we encourage you to seek opportunities to learn MBSR in a class situation.

If you are thinking about enrolling in an MBSR course, our book can give you a sense of what it could be like. In it we discuss both the attitudes that will help you practice mindfulness and how to maintain those attitudes on an everyday basis.

If you are taking part in an MBSR course now, or if you have done so in the past, our book is intended to help you further explore the themes presented in class. It complements the handbook and home practice assignments given out during a course.

If it is not possible for you to take a course, our book will still be helpful as you explore how mindfulness can support you while you live in a way that embodies connection and presence and gain a sense of integration in your daily life.

To begin to practice mindfulness is to embark on a journey that has no end. Mindfulness is not something we "get" and complete. It is a practice for life *and* a lifelong practice. If you take mindfulness to heart, it has the potential to enrich your life in countless ways.

A wise statement from the ancient Chinese tradition of Taoism says, "The path is not the way, the way is the path." Mindfulness informs the way we live with attention, tenderness, and genuine curiosity. It is true strength without force, and true compassion without sentimentality. In a gentle but firm way it says what we already know to be true: the only moment is now! Mindfulness helps us acknowledge the gift of being present in our lives of richness and unfolding possibility.

Life does not have to go our way.
When we know our life is the way,
We can know peace and true fulfillment
That is not dependent on any set of circumstances.

— Linda Lehrhaupt

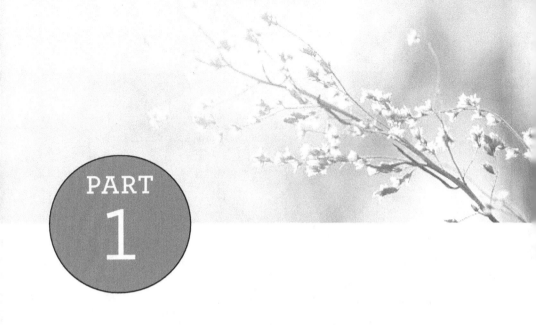

PART 1

Getting Started in MBSR

Background Basics

1

What Is MBSR and Who Can Benefit from It?

Mindfulness-Based Stress Reduction (MBSR) is taught as an eight-week course of usually two-and-a-half- to three-hour sessions, with a full day of silent mindfulness practice between the sixth and seventh meeting. Dr. Jon Kabat-Zinn developed MBSR at the University of Massachusetts Medical Center in Worcester. Inspired by his own experiences with Vipassana and Zen meditation, as well as yoga, Kabat-Zinn taught the first MBSR course in 1979. MBSR was part of the then-emerging field known today as mind-body, or integrative, medicine.

At its core, MBSR is an intensive training in mindfulness, which Kabat-Zinn has defined as "the awareness that arises by paying attention on purpose, in the present moment and non-judgmentally."[1] The most detailed training and study of mindfulness occur in Buddhist traditions, particularly Vipassana, but mindfulness is expressed in other contemplative traditions as well. Since the 1970s it has been integrated into Western health care, education, and other fields and is seen as a nondenominational, nonreligious training available to everyone, whatever their belief. As Kabat-Zinn notes, mindfulness

> is a way of looking deeply into oneself in the spirit of self-inquiry and self-understanding. For this reason it can be learned and practiced, as is done in mindfulness-based programs throughout the world, without appealing to Asian culture or Buddhist authority to enrich it or authenticate it. Mindfulness stands on its own as

3

a powerful vehicle for self-understanding and healing. In fact, one of the major strengths of MBSR and of all other specialized mindfulness-based programs such as mindfulness-based cognitive therapy (MBCT) is that they are not dependent on any belief system or ideology.[2]

Shortly after Kabat-Zinn began teaching MBSR, the Stress Reduction Clinic at the University of Massachusetts Medical Center opened with MBSR as its flagship program. During a one-year trial phase, the clinic held stress-reduction courses with up to thirty participants in each class, many of them chronic-pain patients. The course proved effective in that participants learned to handle their pain in a better way. Their personal suffering diminished, and in some cases their pain levels were reduced in intensity.

From the outset, Kabat-Zinn and his coworkers did research studies.[3] MBSR has been shown to be helpful in reducing symptoms and improving the quality of life for people experiencing a wide range of conditions.

MBSR was the first of what are now known as mindfulness-based interventions or approaches. Programs whose formats (including course length and emphasis on practice at home) are modeled on MBSR include, among others, Mindfulness-Based Cognitive Therapy (MBCT), Mindfulness-Based Eating Awareness Training (MB-EAT), Mindfulness-Based Relapse Prevention (MBRP), and Mindfulness-Based Cancer Care. The main difference between MBSR and these more specialized programs is that the latter generally target people with a specific condition — for example, chronic pain, multiple relapses of depression, substance abuse, cancer, and so on. MBSR courses address participants who have an array of conditions but who are not separated according to their diagnosis or situation.

MBSR is being taught throughout the world by a wide range of professionals, including physicians, psychologists, psychotherapists, schoolteachers, social workers, coaches, physiotherapists, nurses, occupational therapists, chaplains, yoga teachers, and many more people in a wide variety of environments and institutions, including hospitals, psychiatric clinics, universities, private practices, schools, hospices, adult-education institutes, corporations, prisons, counseling centers, medical schools, the armed forces, and many other settings.[4]

MBSR is suitable for people who want to learn to cope with stress using their own resources to improve the quality of their lives. A key element of the course is seeing that it is possible to shift the way we view events or conditions in our lives. In the MBSR course, participants learn that practicing mindfulness can help alleviate their symptoms by creating a wider context for their condition. Rather than focusing on the situation itself, we learn to observe the way we relate to it on emotional, intellectual, and behavioral levels. In the case of relating to pain, for example, some clients in our classes report that the emotional pain (anger, blaming, resignation, a sense of helplessness) they experienced before the course no longer dominates their waking moments. While participating in the course they have practiced being aware of thoughts as thoughts rather than facts, enabling them to create some distance rather than be carried away by them. By practicing the formal MBSR exercises, and particularly the body scan, pain patients can begin to shift their relationship to pain from "I am my pain" to "My body is experiencing pain, but it is not all of me." They may still experience physical pain, but it does not narrow their life choices or dominate their thoughts as much as it did before.

In summing up the relationship between scientific studies and the way we see ourselves, Kabat-Zinn points to the health-enhancing qualities that mindfulness of thoughts and emotions can support:

> If we can be aware — especially *in our own personal experience*, as well as from the evidence from scientific studies — that certain attitudes and ways of seeing ourselves and others are health-enhancing: — that affiliative trust, compassion, kindness, and seeing the basic goodness in others and in ourselves has intrinsic healing power, as does seeing crises and even threats as challenges and opportunities, then we can work mindfully to consciously develop these qualities in ourselves from moment to moment and from day to day. They become new options for us to cultivate. They become new and profoundly satisfying ways of seeing and being in the world.[5]

Who Can Benefit from an MBSR Course?

People enroll in MBSR courses for a variety of reasons. Here are a few typical statements from participants in our classes:

- "When I get stressed, I tend to be dominated by negative thoughts that influence my mood to such an extent that I am no longer capable of being productive. I want to learn to deal with challenges in a calmer and more tranquil way."
- "I would like to develop a better relationship with my body."
- "I want to learn a different approach for coping with stress than the one I've used until now — namely, feeling helpless and paralyzed and blaming others."
- "I take medicine for my illness, and I do what the doctor tells me. But I want to take care of all of me, not just the parts that don't work."
- "I want to get a better sense of my limits and stay in tune with myself. Even when I find it difficult emotionally, I want to be more aware of myself."
- "I want to be aware earlier when stress is building in me and to have the tools to work with it."
- "I want to learn how to stay relaxed even when I'm in stressful situations."
- "What appeals to me about MBSR is that I can learn to take time for myself on a daily basis and to appreciate myself once again."
- "I am looking for something to counterbalance my hectic work life, and I want to learn how to relax again."
- "I want to find better ways of dealing with the minor emergencies of everyday life."
- "I am restricted by chronic pain to such an extent that

it's the only thing on my mind. I want to find a better
way of coping with pain."

- "Until recently I had no problems with stress; in fact, it
was almost as if I needed stress to make me feel good.
But now this doesn't seem to work anymore, and I
don't know what's wrong with me. I seem to be increasingly restless and nervous, and my family says I
am very irritable lately."
- "I work about ten hours a day, and I enjoy it. But I find
it hard to wind down in the evenings. I'm constantly on
the go, and I have the feeling that's not good in the long
run. I want to find a better way to switch off."

Alleviating symptoms of illness and stress is an important aspect of
an MBSR course and an understandable motivation for many to join,
but practicing mindfulness and making it part of our daily lives goes
far beyond reducing the symptoms of an illness. Mindfulness is more
than a problem-solving technique. It is a fundamental shift in attitude
toward ourselves and whatever our condition might be. It helps us tap
into our inner resources and capacities and access the potential for healing that we all have. This in turn creates the basis for an inner orientation toward a wholesome way of life. In this sense, mindfulness is a
fundamental *attitude and way of living.*

Developing a kind and compassionate attitude toward ourselves is
a key factor in the healing power of mindfulness. By *healing*, we do not
mean curing an illness or getting rid of debilitating symptoms. Healing
in this context is related to experiencing wholeness, and we *can* experience a sense of wholeness, even in the midst of serious illness.

Karin, an MBSR course participant who has multiple sclerosis
(MS), speaks of this. She regularly attends MBSR follow-up days offered for former students. She expressed the value of mindfulness practice for her life in the following way: "It's becoming increasingly clear

what the MBSR course did for me in terms of the way I deal with MS. At the beginning of the mindfulness journey, I saw myself as someone who 'suffered' from MS. Thanks to the training I now say: 'I live with MS.' Perhaps this new attitude, and the ability to experience the difference, is the point of mindfulness practice; but for me it is also about the possibility of suffering and living, both at the same time."

A study at Basel University Hospital in Switzerland supports Karin's personal experiences of the benefits of MBSR for her. The study shows that MS patients who took part in an MBSR course experienced more vitality and better quality of life and suffered less frequently from depression.[6]

Which Conditions Does MBSR Help?

In addition to MBSR's preventive and supportive role in helping us cope with everyday stress — at work and at home — scientific studies have shown that it can be helpful in alleviating the symptoms and psychological distress of a range of conditions. These include:

- chronic pain
- cardiovascular diseases (e.g., high blood pressure)
- sleep disorders
- depression and anxiety
- fibromyalgia
- psoriasis
- chronic diseases (e.g., diabetes, multiple sclerosis)
- cancer
- common stress and burnout

There has been an explosion of scientific studies on MBSR and mindfulness-meditation training in recent years. In his pioneering research at the University of Wisconsin, Dr. Richard Davidson documented that mindfulness-meditation training can stimulate neuroplasticity, which he defines as "a capacity of the brain to change its structure and function in significant ways." He goes on to note,

> The amazing fact is that through mental activity alone we can intentionally change our own brains. Mental activity, ranging from meditation to cognitive-behavior therapy, can alter brain function in specific circuits, with the result that you can develop a broader awareness of social signals, a deeper sensitivity to your own feelings and bodily sensations, and a more consistently positive outlook.[7]

In 1999, Dr. Davidson and his team conducted an important study on MBSR. Participants took part in an eight-week MBSR course; a control group did not take part in this class (but was offered the same course when the study was over). Results of the study included a reduction of anxiety symptoms of about 12 percent (as opposed to a slight increase in the control group). According to Dr. Davidson, the MBSR course participants showed that the level of left-side activation of the prefrontal cortex had tripled after four months. This was significant because it reflected "the fact that people practicing this form of mental training learn to redirect their thoughts and feelings[,] ... reducing activity in the negative-emotion right prefrontal cortex and ramping it up in the resilience- and well-being-boosting left side."[8]

All of the study participants, including the control group, were also given a flu shot, and the MBSR students' production of antibodies in response to the vaccine was 5 percent higher than that of the control group. For Davidson this was "an indication that their immune systems responded more effectively than those of the control group."[9]

In the 2013 revised edition of his book *Full Catastrophe Living*, Jon Kabat-Zinn summarized other studies he considered significant for documenting the effects of MBSR.[10] They included the following:

- A study at Massachusetts General Hospital and Harvard University showed that after an eight-week course, density increased in regional gray matter of the brain. These regions, according to Kabat-Zinn, are "associated with learning and memory, emotional regulation, the sense of self, and perspective taking."

• A study at the University of Toronto showed increases in neural activity in a region of the brain associated with experiencing the present moment. At the same time, decreases in the area of the brain known as the "narrative network" were also recorded. According to Kabat-Zinn, "These findings imply that by learning to inhabit the present moment in an embodied way, people can learn how not to get so caught up in the drama of their narrative self, or, for that matter, lost in thought or mind wandering — and when they do get lost in these ways, that they can recognize what is happening and return their attention to what is most salient and important in the present moment."

• A study at UCLA and Carnegie Mellon University showed that loneliness was reduced in a group of participants aged fifty-five to eighty-five who took part in an MBSR course. This is significant because loneliness is one of the emotional states implicated in greater health risks.

MBSR has been shown to be helpful in improving the quality of life and reducing symptoms for people in every age group and in a wide range of conditions. One of the many examples of how MBSR can help a particular section of the population is the improvement of the quality of life for seniors, including those suffering from dementia, as well as for their caregivers. Lucia McBee, who led MBSR groups with elderly people in nursing homes in the United States for more than seven years, reports that following an MBSR course, participants experienced, among other things, pain relief, general well-being, and, in dementia patients, reduced restlessness.[11]

Taking part in an MBSR course also helped caregivers better cope with the double burdens of earning a living and attending to someone who needs care. The same was true for nurses and other staff members in psychiatric hospitals, nursing homes, and acute care clinics. One way MBSR has been helpful for those dealing with occupational stress in general is by teaching people how to be more in touch with themselves and to recognize and respect their own boundaries.

When Would Participation in an MBSR Course Not Be Advisable?

In some situations or conditions, participation in a course is not generally recommended. This includes when a person is actively addicted to a substance or in a state of acute depression. (When participants are stable in a nondepressive phase or have been substance-free for a significant period, MBSR may well be suitable for them.) Taking part in an MBSR course as presented in this book is also contraindicated for those with serious psychiatric disorders such as schizophrenia and psychosis. Clinical trials with mindfulness have been conducted for patients with severe psychiatric disorders; however, this is beyond the scope of our book.

Cancer patients undergoing chemotherapy treatment, and others suffering from severe physical symptoms, may find an MBSR course too physically taxing during their treatment phase. It is advisable for such individuals to wait until their condition is stable enough to permit them to attend class each week and complete the weekly course assignments at home.

Similarly, if you have recently experienced a profound life event, such as the death of a loved one or a life-threatening diagnosis, it may be advisable first to seek support at a counseling center from a psychotherapist or a support group. Once a degree of emotional stability is present, an MBSR course can be a wonderful support for your situation. MBSR is also very helpful as a complement to psychotherapy.

We suggest seeking contact with an MBSR teacher and discussing your personal situation. She or he will be very happy to help you determine whether an MBSR course is an appropriate choice and to assist you in reflecting on your own intentions and motivation.

An intention to participate as fully as possible during the program, and to commit yourself to a healthy and well-balanced lifestyle, is the most important aspect of enrolling in an MBSR course. If you are not personally convinced of the possible value of a course of action, then recommendations or persuasion by others — including well-meaning loved ones, friends, or even your doctor — will not provide the motivation necessary to keep you on track during the course.

What Is the Difference between Mindfulness Practice and Relaxation Methods?

Some participants experience a sense of relaxation while practicing mindfulness of the body or mindfulness of sensations, or while doing other exercises within the MBSR course, but not always. Bringing mindfulness to all areas of our lives — including the difficult ones — can also mean that we are initially more aware of dissatisfaction or stress or pain than we were before, simply because we are turning our attention to these areas. This also explains why, during the early stages of an MBSR course, participants often report that they are more conscious of just how restless their minds actually are and how often they find their thoughts drifting off to the past or future. Some say they are more aware of pain in the body or disturbing thoughts. In truth, mindfulness does not cause more disturbing thoughts or painful sensations. We are simply more attuned and sensitive to these elements, noticing something we were not conscious of before or had been pushing into the background.

A short exercise like the following one on awareness of the body and breath can help illustrate the difference between mindfulness and a relaxation exercise.

Exercise: Awareness of the Body and the Breath

Sit in a comfortable and upright position as best you can, wherever you happen to be at this moment. Then turn your attention to your body. Take some time to feel into your body for the sensations that might be present. If sensations are there, just notice them without trying to change them. If there is any tension in the body, then just allow it to be as it is right now.

Turning your attention to the breath, be with its flow as best you can:

- Sense the body breathing.
- Be aware of the in breath and the out breath and, perhaps, also of the pauses between the breaths.

As you do this exercise, you may notice that your awareness wanders off and you become occupied with ideas, emotions, pictures, or other forms of sensory input. Simply observe when that happens, and then gently and clearly return your awareness to the beginning of the next round of breathing in and breathing out. Continue the exercise for as long as it feels comfortable to you.

If you are new to this practice, we suggest that you experiment with doing it for five minutes a day to begin with. You may also practice at various times during the day for shorter periods, and do so seated, standing, or lying down.

When we do exercises like "Awareness of the Body and the Breath," a question the MBSR teacher might ask afterward is: "What did you experience?" You probably noticed while doing the exercise that your thoughts jumped to other objects or activities several times, perhaps continually. This is entirely normal and shows, in fact, how little our attention is anchored in the present moment. This is precisely what we need to observe at the outset of our practice: *the mind is often restless.*

If we are intent on achieving relaxation, we may instead find that we have tightened up or become sharply focused on the breath. This can lead to shortness of breath or other physical symptoms related to tension. We may then sense that we have failed to do the exercise properly, as well as feel disappointed that relaxation has not occurred.

If we see this as a mindfulness exercise, we practice noticing the breath and anything else that might occur, including our intention to relax or our attempt to physically control our breathing. If we notice we are tense, we stay with exactly what we experience (sensations, thoughts, emotions) as best we can, without trying to change anything. We are focused not on results but on what is happening from moment to moment.

Practicing mindfulness may create a sense of relaxation, but that is different from having a fixed goal of achieving relaxation. The interesting thing is that, whatever comes up simply as an event that is happening, tension is often no longer such an issue and, with time, can lose its stress-provoking effect.

Mindfulness practice involves allowing ourselves to feel whatever is present in the moment. This attitude is wholesome — and possibly relaxing — for the mind as well as the body.

2 What Is Mindfulness?

Simply put, mindfulness is moment-to-moment non-judgmental awareness. It is cultivated by purposefully paying attention to things we ordinarily never give a moment's thought to. It is a systematic approach to developing new kinds of agency, control, and wisdom in our lives, based on our inner capacity for paying attention and on the awareness, insight, and compassion that naturally arise from paying attention in specific ways.[12]

— Jon Kabat-Zinn, *Full Catastrophe Living*

We'd like to draw your attention to some key aspects of Jon Kabat-Zinn's above description of mindfulness. We refer to these elements in different ways throughout the book, especially in the mindfulness exercises in MBSR.

- *Mindfulness takes place in the present moment.* We are rarely in the present moment. When we're lost in memories of the past or anticipation of the future, we often become caught up in a way that hijacks our attention, making it more difficult to stay in the everyday moments of our lives.

- *Mindfulness can be trained and strengthened.* The practice of mindfulness can be compared to muscle-strengthening exercises. In much the same way that our muscles can weaken or atrophy when not exercised, our capacity for mindfulness can weaken or atrophy when we don't make use of it. The core of MBSR is the systematic training of the muscle of mindfulness.

- *Mindfulness can be cultivated.* When we practice mindfulness, we tend the garden of our life, watering and caring for it. Everything nourishes this garden: the wonderful moments of our lives as well as the difficult ones. The difficult ones in particular — what one meditation teacher called the "compost of our lives" — can provide a rich source of nourishment as we learn to meet them with mindfulness.

- *In mindfulness training, we strengthen our capacity for nonjudgmental awareness.* One of the first things we notice as we practice mindfulness is how caught up we are in judgments, ideas, and opinions about things and our lives in general. As we continue to practice mindfulness, we see that it is possible to set judging aside (at least some of the time) and experience elements of our lives in a less-filtered way, freer of tunnel vision. This may in turn create a richer and clearer understanding that we have a choice about things. Opting to exercise that choice becomes a conscious step toward mindful action, rather than a detour into wishful thinking, resignation, or impulsive behavior.

- *Mindfulness gives us access to our own wisdom, insight, and compassion.* If we reverse the syllables in the word *insight*, it reads as "sight in," which means "sight within ourselves." Mindfulness develops our capacity to look inward and access the rich ground of wisdom of our lives.

What Mindfulness Meditation Is Not

- Mindfulness meditation is not a journey of the imagination that encourages us to abandon ourselves to fantasies.
- It is not a relaxation exercise. Although we may experience a sense of relaxation during and after practice, relaxation is not the goal.
- Mindfulness meditation is not about escaping from the world and our everyday reality. In MBSR we practice exactly the opposite — being aware of the present moment just as it is, even if it is painful.
- It is not a quest for alternative states of consciousness or about developing out-of-the-ordinary mental or physical capacities.
- Mindfulness meditation is not about making our minds blank, although it is a popular misconception that blankness is the goal.

The Whole World in a Raisin:
The Experience of Mindfulness

We can talk about mindfulness, but ultimately the reality of mindfulness is the experience of it. That's why we'd like to give you an opportunity to experience mindfulness with a mindful eating exercise. It is the same exercise that tens of thousands of people have taken part in since the founding of MBSR in 1979.

You can read the instructions and do the exercise by yourself; but if you can, it's helpful to have someone read them to you. Another option is to make an audio recording of the exercise. Whatever you choose, remember: *really* eating is not the same as reading about it.

It is a tradition in MBSR to use raisins for this exercise. If you don't like raisins, we encourage you to try the exercise with them anyway. Often in an MBSR class, people who haven't eaten raisins for many years decide to do so for this exercise. Later in the chapter we'll share what some of them have had to say about their experiences.

If you are allergic to raisins, perhaps you can use another dried fruit.

Mindful Eating Exercise 1: Our Five Senses

We invite you to place three raisins in front of you on a clean surface. Imagine that you have never seen these objects (we'll call them this from now on) before, and you don't know what they are. You will be using each of your five senses (sight, hearing, touch, smell, and taste) to investigate them. If one of these senses is not available to you, imagine what it might be like if you did have that sense.

Please take a moment to pause and note your experience as you move through each phase — and sense — of the exercise. We'll make some suggestions, but please feel free to explore whatever arises for you.

The Sense of Sight

Pick up one object and examine it carefully. Imagine you are describing it to someone over the telephone. What would you say about its surface? What color is it? Is there more than one color?

Is it shiny, dull, or both? Are there lines on its surface? Are they wavy, straight, both? What happens when you hold the object up to the light? Can you see through it? Is there anything inside? What else have you noticed?

The Sense of Touch

Rub the object between your fingers. How would you describe its surface? Is it rough or smooth? Wet, dry, or sticky? Does it feel swollen? Is it thick or thin? Is it stretchy or brittle? What else comes to mind about the way it feels?

The Sense of Hearing

What does the object sound like? We suggest raising it up to one ear and rubbing it between your fingers. What do you hear? Is it a sharp or dull sound, if anything? Is it loud or soft? Are there other words that describe the sound you hear?

Move the object to the other ear. What do you hear now? Is it the same sound or a different one? Is it softer or louder?

The Sense of Smell

Hold the object under your nose. How would you describe its smell? Is it sharp? Acrid? Bitter? Oily? Sweet? Musty?

Press down on one nostril to close it, smelling the object through the other nostril. Then, switch nostrils. Does the smell vary on each side? Is there a difference in intensity? Move the object back and forth a few times between nostrils, just smelling.

The Sense of Taste

Move the object to your mouth and try outlining your lips with it, as if it were lipstick. Do you notice anything? Are there sensations inside the mouth as well as outside? How would you describe them?

Now place the object in your mouth. Don't bite down, but use your tongue to explore its surface. Try rolling it inside your mouth, pressing it against your gums. Try placing it under your tongue. Continue, as best you can, to be aware of the sensations inside your mouth as the object sits or moves within it. Does the object stay firm? Does it soften or even seem to melt?

Now place the object between your back teeth on one side of

your mouth. Sense it resting between your molars. Are you aware of any intentions or impulses? Do you experience an urge to bite down?

When you are ready, bite down and chew as slowly as you can, softly grinding the fruit between your teeth. Notice the flavors that are released. How would you describe them? Continue chewing slowly until every bit of the object has disappeared.

Preparing to swallow, notice the intention as it arises. As you swallow, notice if you can sense the movement at the back of your throat, then farther down, as far as you can go.

Are there any traces of the object left in your mouth? Is there still a taste present, though there is no object? Take time to be with whatever sensations, thoughts, or emotions may be present.

Mindful Eating Exercise 2: Going Deeper

Repeat the exercise on your own without any guidance. Explore the second object in the same way as you did with the first, using each of the five senses: sight, touch, hearing, smell, and taste. Take the time you need, and be aware of any tendencies or impulses to speed up, slow down, or drift off into thought as you engage in this mindful eating exercise.

When we teach this exercise in an MBSR class, people move through the exercise at their own pace. Some are long finished when others are just beginning to chew on the object.

Mindful Eating Exercise 3: Just Eating

Just eat the third object the way you normally would. Notice how you place it in your mouth. Do you pop it in quickly? Do you chew rapidly or slowly? Were you even aware of chewing? Like many participants in our classes, you may find yourself chuckling at this point.

A Moment of Reflection

We invite you to take a moment to reflect on these objects, which are of course raisins. They are dried grapes, which can grow in the wild but are usually farmed in areas where it is hot during the summer. The fields where they are cultivated may be hilly or flat. They need a considerable amount of sun to ripen and even more to dry out. Picture the vines or branches heavy with fruit at harvest time.

There are countless people who have had direct or indirect contact with your raisins. Someone planted the vines, watered the fields, harvested them either by machine or by hand, loaded them into containers, and arranged to transport them. Someone packaged them and someone else placed the package on a shelf in the store, where you bought it.

There is a whole web of people and places connected to your three raisins. Please take some time to reflect on this. Notice what arises as you have a sense of how all life and living itself is connected and in relationship.

What the Raisin Exercise Tells Us about Our Lives and How We Relate to Them

Here are some of the most frequent comments that our course participants make about the mindful eating exercise. We would also like to show how these comments relate to some key aspects of mindfulness and its role in our everyday lives.

> *I had no idea a raisin looks the way it does.*
> *And each of them is completely different.*

Each object in the world is unique. Even machine-made objects have tiny differences. Appreciating uniqueness is an important shift in awareness. Rather than reducing everything to sameness, we celebrate individuality as we become more mindful. This applies not only to raisins but also to everything around us: people, places, and the stars in an evening sky.

Yet how often do we look at something and think we have seen it before? How often do we touch something and think we know what it feels like?

When we are living with the pressure of deadlines, illness, or physical pain, or in any number of situations where we feel stressed, life can become flat, colorless, and repetitive. The possibility of seeing different perspectives sharply diminishes, and we lose the sense that life is varied. We resent change rather than accept its potential for richness. We seek sameness and long for routine.

Making a conscious decision to look deeply and with fresh eyes, without knowing exactly what we will find, is a vital step in practicing mindfulness. It is often referred to as "beginner's mind," a term coined by Shunryu Suzuki, a pioneering Japanese Zen master who taught in San Francisco from 1959 until his death in 1971. We could also call this attitude of looking with freshness "baby mind," because mindfulness encourages us to explore new objects (and experiences) with all of our senses, just the way a baby does. Zen Buddhist teacher Darlene Cohen, who wrote with deep compassion about living with chronic pain, calls it "puppy mind," referring to the way puppies joyfully explore an object when it is new to them.[13]

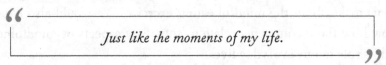

Just like the moments of my life.

Emily was diagnosed with breast cancer and had a radical mastectomy. After radiation treatment, she was able to return to work and take up her life again. Seven years later, some pimples on her chest were the first signs that the cancer had returned. She decided to try MBSR after a round of chemotherapy was over. At her preinterview for the MBSR class, she said, "I don't know how long I have to live...but in a film I heard someone say something like, 'You want to go from existing to living.'" Emily paused and then added with determination: "And that's what I want to learn, too!"

When the class shared their experiences with each other after the raisin exercise, Emily took her time before she spoke. When she did, her voice was full of joy. "I always thought I knew what raisins tasted like, but now I know that they can have many different tastes. Just like the moments of my life. How wonderful!"

Emily's delight illustrates how mindfulness can help us celebrate the infinite variety of life. Even when facing a difficult prognosis, Emily was able to savor what she came to call "life's precious moments."

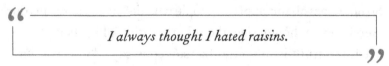

I always thought I hated raisins.

The key word in this comment is *thought*. When we apply an opinion formed in the past to something in the present, the past rules our lives. It controls what we experience and what we don't. It obscures the present with shadows of things that have already occurred. It's not *now*; it's *then*.

In the mindful eating exercise, we may decide not to taste the raisin because we don't like it. Perhaps we didn't like it in the past, but what about now? Can we really know whether we like it or not at this time without tasting it?

The consequences of refusing to try something in the present because we made a decision about it in the past may not be a big deal as far as raisins are concerned. But what about all the other things we have cut out of our lives? Perhaps we don't go to a certain place because we once had a disagreeable experience there, or perhaps we avoid certain people, or won't apply for a certain kind of job, or made a decision long ago that we would never have the hip replacement our doctor recommended and we are now in a lot of pain. Or...or...or...

The consequences of frozen-in-time opinions are no different for things we like. We seek out the things with which we have a pleasant association. If we go to dinner and there is a choice between something we like and something unfamiliar, the chances are good we will pick the food we like. If we are used to dressing a certain way, we tend to buy clothes like the ones we usually wear.

There is nothing wrong with knowing what we like and what we don't. At the same time, it is helpful to be conscious of the consequences of how likes and dislikes affect our choices and actions. Simply put, the more unaware we are of how much our likes and dislikes filter, control, and shape our world, the more we restrict ourselves. Not out of choice but out of habit.

So how does all this apply to people who decide to eat raisins during the exercise even though they thought they didn't like them?

Well, the truth is, it's rare that someone says, "Oh, you know, I really like raisins now!" Nevertheless, what participants often say is: "Raisins taste different than what I thought."

A teacher of Korean Zen Buddhism, Seung Sahn Sunim (1927–2004), was famous for continually reminding his students: "Only don't know!" And his answer to many questions was: "Keep don't-know mind!" When we practice mindfulness, we cultivate a spirit of not-knowing. It is not that we know nothing; rather, keeping don't-know mind encourages a willingness to meet whatever is before us without preconditions or preconceived ideas. We try to experience it as it is, not as we think it is.

Likes and dislikes are habits of the mind.
They feel real because they are familiar.
Mindfulness brings each moment to life.
We can be aware of uniqueness or sameness and not be caught
   in either.

— Linda Lehrhaupt

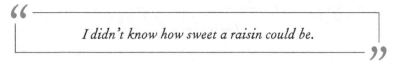

> *I didn't know how sweet a raisin could be.*

The level of sweetness they taste during the raisin exercise often surprises class participants. For some, the flavor explodes in their mouths with the first bite. For others, it becomes most apparent as they eat a second or third raisin. Almost always someone says, "I rarely have this intensity when I eat. How much have I been missing from my food?" Invariably the question that follows is: "What am I missing in my life?"

This realization — that we miss so many moments of life — can make us feel sorrow, anger, puzzlement, renewed determination, and a host of other sentiments. A sense of having lost opportunities might overwhelm us: friends gone, youth lost, bad choices. The same awareness can awaken a commitment to honor life's moments — indeed, to value them as precious — not with a sense of loss or having to cling to them, but with the same wakefulness with which we savored each raisin.

Many MBSR class participants come to realize that the more they are in touch with all aspects of their lives, the more alive they feel. In the past, they may have been afraid of being overwhelmed or hurt and so avoided certain situations. One participant described the impulse to dodge a feeling as a need "to raise the drawbridge to my heart."

Many glimpse in the mindful eating exercise, and during the weeks that follow, that when they are present for the rich field of sensations and experiences that they encounter from moment to moment, life is no longer the same. Life shifts and unfolds in myriad ways.

We begin to discover resilience and vitality when we are no longer so guarded. We learn to trust that we will know what needs to be done. When we decide to shift direction or make a choice, the strength of that trust allows us to raise or lower the drawbridge of our hearts, not in panic, but mindfully.

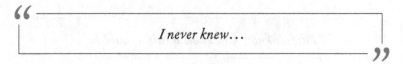

I never knew...

The following MBSR class participants began to describe their experiences with the raisin exercise by saying, "I never knew" and then went on to say how it related to something in their lives.

Heike, whose husband, Frank, had recently died of cancer, expressed sadness. She shared how sorry she was that she had never taken enough time off from work when Frank was alive to enjoy their garden or the meals he loved to cook. She put her career first and was often away on long business trips, even after her husband's diagnosis of prostate cancer. She told us that she never knew how precious her life with Frank had been until he was gone.

Jürgen felt gratitude. Now forty-two, he had suffered from Crohn's disease since he was a teenager. He mentioned the long years of struggle and pain brought on by his illness. Forced to retire early, he had begun to do things he'd never had time for, including paying more attention to his diet and nurturing his friendships. During the raisin exercise, he realized he "never knew" how rich his life was, because he once thought that the only thing of real value in his life was the work he had had to give up.

Gertrude, too, felt a deep sense of loss. She had enrolled in an MBSR course, she said, because of the stress she suffered from breaking contact with her adult son following a family dispute. In class she exhibited a sharp energy, as if she were determined to always get everything right. During the raisin exercise her eyes filled with tears. She told us, "I thought I made the right decision by cutting him off. I never knew I'd lost the most precious thing I ever had... my relationship with my son."

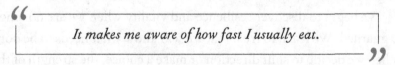

It makes me aware of how fast I usually eat.

Slowing down to eat a raisin with as much focus and intent as we do in an MBSR class is almost a revolutionary act. How it differs from the way we normally consume food becomes even more evident with the second raisin. On our own, without guidance, our tendency is to speed up: but for almost everyone in class, even then, eating takes much longer than usual.

Sometimes I (Linda) tell my classes about the slow food movement, a worldwide network of people who take pleasure in preparing and savoring sustainable foods and regional recipes. The emphasis is on fresh, locally grown, unprocessed foods and taking time to eat together.

When I first moved to Germany in 1983 to live with my husband, Norbert, he was amazed when, on the very first morning after I arrived, I said, "Let's go out for breakfast."

"But why should we do that?" he asked. "We have everything here that we need. I'll just go get some fresh bread." Before I could say another word, he was out the door and on his way to the bakery.

It took me quite some time to break the habit of breakfast on the run. I was used to eating out — and quickly — in New York City. Meals at home with my husband and the many other Europeans I came to know over the years became a celebration in the slow-food way. Of course, we went out to dinner sometimes, but those occasions became special because I no longer took them for granted.

There's a truly delightful film about the joy of tasting food called *Babette's Feast*. It teaches a lesson about food and pleasure that can make even the most die-hard "bagel-to-go" New Yorker take stock, stop, and savor. The story is about a chef who worked at one of the most famous restaurants in Paris in the late eighteenth century. She was forced to flee to Denmark during the French Revolution and was given refuge and employment by two staunchly Calvinist spinsters. They were unaware of their cook's narrow escape and how she had lost her husband and son in the turmoil. The sisters ask her to prepare a memorial dinner for their father, a stern pastor who had died the year before. Normally admonished to cook simply, Babette decides to show her appreciation to the sisters by cooking a sumptuous French feast and paying for it herself. The film chronicles the making and consuming of a slow-food dinner of the most joyful and sensuous kind. As the guests become overwhelmed by their own joy and sense of taste, they allow their humanity to surface.

> "
> *It's like I'm on automatic pilot.*
> *I was chewing before I even realized it.*
> "

During the mindful eating exercise, many people become aware of how hard it is not to bite down on the raisin. Some forget the instruction not to chew and are munching away before they realize it.

In MBSR we refer to remaining unaware while engaging in an activity as "being on automatic pilot." Many of us experience this while driving a car. Sometimes we leave home and arrive at our destination with no recollection of the time in between. We may have been absorbed in a radio program or just "out to lunch," but who knows what we missed while we tuned out?

There is a downside to living as if on automatic pilot. Many people operate this way, going through the motions with their families or coworkers with no sense of real connection. Consider our work lives — pressures can keep people busy and even productive but leave less time for human interaction and impart a sense of lost community. The stages of the life cycle — birth, maturation, and death, for example — can become inconvenient events rather than life passages worthy of our attention and celebration.

It is possible to awaken attention, to become aware of not being aware. This is a key aspect of mindfulness training. To notice when we're either lost in thought or multitasking without doing one thing completely is to be mindful. When we are mindful, it is possible to restore our awareness and liveliness — our presence in the present.

When we are aware that we are not there, we are right here, right now.
When we are aware that we are not aware, we are practicing mindfulness.

— Linda Lehrhaupt

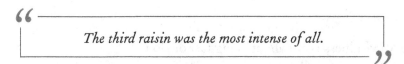

The third raisin was the most intense of all.

This comment brings up an interesting point about the relationship between rushing and mindfulness. In the third part of the exercise, people eat the raisin in the way that many people normally do, which usually means popping it into their mouths and swallowing, often with only minimal chewing. If that's the case, then why do some people report that eating the third raisin is the most intense experience of all?

It is true that slowing down is an important part of learning mindfulness. It allows us to savor all the aspects of an experience in a more tactile way. It also gives us an opportunity to be aware of an experience moment to moment. In MBSR we encourage participants to practice all the exercises slowly. If we engage in an everyday activity like washing the dishes or brushing our teeth as a mindfulness exercise at home, slowing down is one of the practice parameters...and it's often what participants find to be the most difficult.

Sometimes we have to move fast — to avoid danger or to save a life. There are many professions where people have to be quick — for example, firefighters, police officers, and emergency room doctors and nurses. How can mindfulness help individuals like these, for whom a few seconds can mean the difference between life and death? How can mindfulness help us engage in sports or in any other situation where speed is a factor?

Mindfulness training applies wonderfully to these situations. Many people who practice mindfulness report that when they have to move quickly, they feel more grounded and aware of the space around them.

We may not all work at jobs where speed is a requirement, but everyone encounters situations when they're under pressure to act quickly. In times of haste, the key aspect is to *connect to what is going on.* By practicing mindfulness, we stay better connected to ourselves and to the situation.

> Mindfulness is not about being fast or slow.
> It is a matter of how we pay attention.
> We can live at the speed of life and remain connected and present.
>
> — Linda Lehrhaupt

" *All we are doing is eating raisins. How extraordinary!* "

There is nothing mysterious about mindfulness. Each of us can describe times when we have experienced it, though we may not have called it mindfulness. It might have been as our child was being born, or during a moment of physical challenge, or when we were negotiating a hairpin turn on a mountain road. It might have been when we watched a sunrise or stood by as a loved one took her last breath.

What do all these moments have in common? They are moments when mindfulness occurs spontaneously. There is a sense of immediacy, of being awake and aware, of clarity. These occasions are often very special, and we tend to remember them with gratitude as extraordinary gifts that life has given us. Yet it is important not to reserve mindfulness only for special moments. Every moment has its unique quality, its essence, and its changing shape. These qualities are present whether we call them "good" or "bad." Maintaining connection to the present gives color, depth, and a celebratory quality to our lives, no matter what the situation. It allows us to experience both the ordinary and the extraordinary as rich moments of our lives.

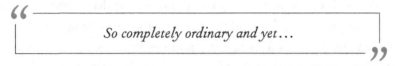

So completely ordinary and yet...

Amy shared with us the deep emotional healing she experienced with her estranged mother, Adele, as she fed her during the last days before she died.

"Mom could eat only the softest foods, like yogurt and apple-sauce. Sometimes it would take me an hour to feed her a small dish. I was so focused on getting the food onto the spoon, holding it near her mouth, waiting for her to find the strength to take a bit in. I lost all sense of time. Life became just one spoonful... and the next... and the next, each spoonful a process of complete giving, acceptance, and letting go. It was so completely ordinary. I thank God that I had the chance to perform such a small task of love. It was a gift of grace."

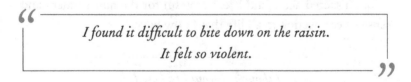

I found it difficult to bite down on the raisin.
It felt so violent.

At least one person in almost every class makes this comment. And then the whole class explores what it is about biting down that could feel aggressive. For many participants it's the fact that they've become aware of all the places the raisin has been and the people who have been in contact with it, which then makes each raisin special. A raisin is no longer anonymous.

What often happens — and this is especially true when we are overwhelmed in life — is that we come to treat other people, ani-mals, and our natural world as mere objects. Once they have become depersonalized, it is easier to misuse, abuse, and deplete them. Sadly, the object we most often treat this way is our own body.

We tend to treat our bodies like machines. Either they function well and we ignore them, or, if we are ill, we judge them as having failed us. We work to the point of burnout and eat or drink ourselves into forgetfulness, yet we discount the harm that we are doing to ourselves. We turn away from life-sustaining relationships and are caught up in acquiring surplus for the sake of surplus, working more hours, sleeping less, and eventually drowning in our own activities. Whether we will look in on our children before they go to sleep, for example, or get that last email of the day answered, becomes a toss-up.

One lesson that the raisin exercise teaches us is that all lives, including our own, are treasures. Our inherent kindness and generosity can be nourished, and in this state of nourishment, true abundance is possible, as is deep kindness to others and ourselves. Maria expressed it this way:

> I found it difficult to bite down on the raisin. It felt so violent. At first I had to force myself to bite down. But when I ate the second raisin, I realized that when I eat with full attention, I can bite down not as an act of violence, but in communion. Eating becomes a sacred act...and I feel grateful for the nourishment and sense of connection to all life that I now have.

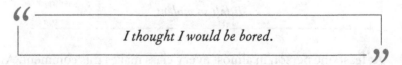

> " *I thought I would be bored.* "

When someone makes this comment, one of the first questions I (Linda) always ask is: "So *were* you bored?" Often the person answers, "No, not while I was doing it. Only when I thought about it beforehand."

During the exercise, participants talk about boredom in different ways. Günther said, "I felt bored during the second and third raisin. Not while the exercise was being guided." John noted, "Well, I was thinking that this exercise was not very interesting. I mean, like: 'I don't have the time for this.'" Maria added, "I've eaten raisins so many times. I worried I'd find it completely boring to have to look at each one." Bruno was somewhat exasperated when he told the class: "I came here to learn how to deal with my physical pain. Not eat raisins. This exercise is stupid."

What we label as boredom is a state where we are sometimes restless and not paying attention in the present moment. It can also feel like an absence of attention, as if there is nothing worth paying attention to. In fact, when we are bored, we are often caught up in thoughts. We may be thinking about the past or the future. We may think we know what we are going to see because we've seen it before. We've disconnected from what is going on right now.

We can become aware of a sense of boredom and use it as a wake-up call, one that tells us when we are withdrawing from whatever is happening. Then, rather than dwelling in boredom, we can raise a sense of curiosity about what is happening in that moment.

When you experience boredom, try to investigate that state completely. As we did with the raisin, turn your attention to whatever is present for you, directly in front of you. Try asking:

"Where is my attention right now?"
"What am I thinking about?"
"What am I sensing?"

In being mindful you can experience a sense of being present in your own life, in contact from moment to moment with your body/mind, as well as with your thoughts, feelings, and sensations. Mindfulness is not a state of awareness that arises only in special situations. In practicing mindfulness, we learn to be aware, and we learn that it is possible to be aware of the moments when we are not aware.

Mindfulness allows us to know where we are and what we're doing, to be at home in our own bodies in the midst of both joy and turmoil.

3

Stress, Life's Challenges, and Mindfulness

In this chapter we consider three basic questions:

- What is stress?
- How is it triggered?
- What are the effects of stress on our quality of life?

Along the way we'll look at how practicing mindfulness helps us work with stress in a beneficial way. We, the authors, feel it makes sense to understand what stress is before we go on to look at how we can learn a wholesome way of living with it. To begin exploring this theme, we invite you to participate in the following exercise based on one developed by Professor Gert Kaluza, one of Germany's leading experts on stress.

Exercise: Exploring Stress Triggers and Stress Reactions

Complete this sentence: "I feel stressed when..."

- Write down whatever comes to mind. It can be one thing or a long list of any conditions or situations in which you feel stressed.
- Next complete this phrase: "When I am stressed, I tend to..." Write down what you do when you experience stress. For example: "I smoke more...I feel helpless

and useless...I am irritable...I go jogging." In this way you can discover your individual reactions to stress triggers.

- Now that you have taken note of your reactions to stress triggers, ask yourself which level you tend primarily to react on:

  - mental-emotional level ("I'm worried," "I can't cope," "It's all too much for me," etc.)
  - physical level (rapid heartbeat, frequent urge to urinate, agitation, etc.)
  - behavioral level (smoking, hyperactivity, etc.)

- Your stress reactions may well include several of these elements.

- You may find that during this exercise you describe obvious, everyday things that trigger stress. These might include: shopping after a long day at work, trying to concentrate in distracting situations, being rushed when there are many small things to take care of, or several people wanting something from you at the same time.

I (Petra) feel stressed when I am faced with a challenging task and can't find a quiet time to work on it because there are so many other things to do. It can also be stressful for me when I am working under a deadline or I have little control over the situation.

It's not only the big, dramatic things — the so-called critical life events, such as marriage, the death of a loved one, or the loss of a job — that generate stress. It's also the ordinary and frequently recurring situations or problems that gnaw at our nerves. Time pressure, excessive demands, or environmental factors such as noise, limited space, or general sensory overload often compound these problems. The findings of stress researchers confirm this: the so-called daily hassles constitute the biggest challenge for our stress-coping skills and therefore the greatest health risk.

You can think of your daily stress factors as grains of sand accumulating in the gears of a machine. Initially they may not affect things too much, but if they're left unattended, real problems can develop for the gears and for our lives. Then, when we're overwhelmed, something minor like a phone ringing or a simple question from a workmate can become a stress trigger, bringing on an intense physical or emotional reaction. It's the proverbial straw that breaks the camel's back.

It doesn't have to be this way. An important aspect of MBSR is learning to practice mindfulness in everyday life so that we maintain an attitude of wakefulness. We also cultivate friendliness toward ourselves so that we can return to the present moment gently, without recrimination. This in turn supports us and helps us recognize early warning signals instead of becoming caught up in an automatic reaction. For example, the exercise on stress triggers above shows us how to spot the warning signs of stress, which helps us avoid getting caught up in them. Mindfulness can also help us pause and ask, "What am I actually feeling at this moment? What is my body telling me about the emotions I am experiencing?" In this way, we can learn to meet stress triggers and reactions with awareness, reducing our tendency to switch to automatic pilot and go through the motions, while not being truly present mentally or emotionally. Later we will see how practicing mindfulness in this way can be helpful in dealing with challenging situations.

When I Reach My Goal, Then I'll Be Happy…Won't I?

This statement reflects an attitude that governs many people's lives. We often focus our attention as well as our hopes on promises of happiness or the big events in our lives. As a result, we tend to lose sight of the subtle, chronic stress this attitude causes. We allow our lives to be dominated — more or less unconsciously — by a "when-then" attitude: "When the children have left home, then I'll take more time for myself " or "When I've finished this project, then things will quiet down." We try to convince ourselves that we will be happier once we have a new car or a new partner, or once we have taken that beach vacation. This attitude is fostered and reinforced by modern society, which supports the notion that contentment lies in status symbols, an attractive physical appearance, success, and wealth — and that these things are more important than serenity, relaxation, our quality of life, and ethics. Australian writer and philosopher Father Alfred D'Souza puts it concisely: "For a long time it seemed to me that life was about to begin — real life. But there was always some obstacle in the way, something to be gotten through first, some unfinished business, time to still be served, a debt to be paid. Then life would begin. At last it dawned on me that these obstacles were my life."[14] The when-then attitude is a stress trigger that fosters the expectation that we can achieve something that might never happen. Living in the future causes us to miss the present.

If we are caught up in a stressful life situation and don't think we can change it, we often think we have no alternative but to accept it. Or we become so accustomed to the stress that we believe we need it to function. Often we end up merely reacting to circumstances instead of taking charge of our lives. All of these situations can lead to living for the weekend or a dream vacation — hoping for some kind of relief. Then, when the vacation or weekend is over, the relaxation we may have experienced soon dissipates. In fact, an irony of modern life is that the leisure we long for does not help us truly relax but instead becomes another source of stress.

Since "doing nothing" is seldom considered a worthwhile objective in our society, many people pack as many "leisure activities" as possible into their "relaxing" weekend. Sometimes we harbor the unexpressed attitude that "the more I do to relax, the more stress-free I will be." By the start of each workweek, we may find that activities such as watching television, going to the movies, dining out, engaging in competitive sports, or going to theme parks or parties have not resulted in true relaxation. We may have been distracted from our concerns, but we have not really coped with stress in a helpful way, by winding down. In fact, we have substituted one sort of stressful activity for another, which may be a distraction from our more accustomed activities but is still an activity that keeps us very much in "doing mode." However, please don't misunderstand us: we are not saying that no one should engage in leisure activities such as those mentioned above, only that it all depends on how we approach them.

Recovering from Stress

Studies on the dynamics of physical stress and relaxation have shown that every stress and exertion phase must be followed by a rest and relaxation phase in order to avoid damage to our health. At the same time, the length of the rest phase depends on the type of stress and its duration. The longer a stress phase lasts, the longer it takes for us to recover and be ready to enter the next stress period with the requisite motivation and ability. Yet most people's daily lives do not allow for this. Either they don't rest at all, or they don't rest enough to provide the necessary amount of relaxation and regeneration before a new phase of activity.

It is important to choose recreational activities that are truly relaxing. Most helpful is a regeneration activity that leads to our feeling better and helps us unwind mentally. Often this is not what happens even when we lie down to rest. Our bodies may be prostrate, but our minds are still busy with plans, worries, or daydreams, and we are far from truly relaxing. The slowing down of mental activity is an essential element for effective recovery, and that is exactly what we practice in mindfulness meditation.

Mindfulness meditation is also about developing a nonjudgmental approach to observing our thoughts and feelings. In doing so, we can avoid getting lost in the litanies of thoughts that are often a major cause of stress and discomfort.

The following exercise may help you understand what we mean by observing our thoughts as thoughts. When this exercise is finished, take a moment to notice what struck you as particularly interesting or new, and what you experienced as you observed your thoughts. Don't worry if you were not able to observe your thoughts at all times. That is normal. Just try repeating the exercise another time. Becoming aware of thoughts in a less stressful way takes quite a bit of practice.

Exercise: Observing Our Thoughts

- First, adopt a comfortable, relaxed, and upright posture while sitting on a chair, sofa, bed, meditation cushion, or bench. Be aware of your posture and the sensations, if any, that are present in the body. Perhaps you sense the parts of your body that are in direct contact with the surface you are sitting on. Then, without changing your position, allow yourself to become aware of your body as a whole. Take some time to notice any sensations that may be present, or simply notice the whole body as it is. Spend about two minutes doing this.

- Now, tune in to the breath and become aware of the fact that your body is breathing. While doing this, you don't need to change anything. For example, there is no need to try to control your breath, to make it deeper or change it in any other way. Give yourself a few moments just to sense your breathing as best you can: inhaling…exhaling…one breath following the other. If you have trouble simply sensing the breath and tend to try to control your breathing, then be gently aware of this. Just sit and continue to practice mindfulness of your breathing for about two minutes.

- Still seated and breathing naturally, begin noticing the

thoughts that arise. If you find this difficult, imagine you are sitting in a movie theater watching an empty screen and waiting for your thoughts to be projected onto it. When these thoughts appear, simply observe them, and then notice what happens if you don't intervene. Some thoughts will disappear as soon as you become aware of them. Others will remain or recur. Just continue to be aware of them as simply thoughts or "mind events," and watch as they appear on the screen and then disappear, without trying to influence them or get involved in their content. If the suggestion of sitting in a movie theater is not helpful, feel free to choose a different image — for instance, observing clouds drifting by in the sky as your thoughts. Or you might want to picture yourself sitting by a river and watching your thoughts float past as if they are boats.

- When you feel ready, bring the exercise to a close by returning your attention to your body while sitting. You may feel like stretching or taking a few deep breaths.
- In observing thoughts, we take a step backward and simply observe them without getting tangled up in them. When you experience this even for a few seconds, you have interrupted the tendency to go on automatic pilot and are deepening your mindfulness practice.

To summarize, the exercise consists of three steps:

1. Adopt a comfortable seated position and become aware of your body.
2. Turn your attention to your breath and be aware of the sensations of breathing.
3. Observe the flow of thoughts without letting yourself be drawn into them.

What Is Stress?

In science there is no single definition of the word *stress*. In everyday usage, the word generally points to mental or physical strain or discomfort. Some people claim they never experience stress, implying that everything in their lives runs smoothly. Often, however, people play down the effect of stress on their lives, because being stressed has largely negative connotations in our society. If we feel stressed, we often say, "I'm stressed out," meaning there are circumstances in our lives that trigger stress. Sometimes we say something like: "My job is really stressful," which describes an experience that is demanding too much of us — an external stress factor. Some people take a certain pride in their stress because it gives them a sense of being busy and important.

Dr. Hans Selye, a Canadian-Hungarian endocrinologist whom many consider the father of stress theory, first defined *stress* in 1936 as "the non-specific response of the body to any demand for change." Based on his numerous studies of the physiological changes in injured animals, he coined the term *stress trigger* (or stressor). Stressors include all external and internal factors that represent a potential threat, including physical pain and difficult emotions. If we are confronted with a stress trigger, it activates the so-called stress reaction. This response follows a specific pattern, as we will see later.

Stress Triggers

Stress triggers vary from person to person, and anything is a potential stress trigger. They include:

- *physiological factors*: pain, disability, illness, hunger, thirst, and symptoms such as heart palpitations or a bloated stomach
- *environmental factors*: excessive cold, noise, heat, and other natural phenomena
- *work-related factors*: deadlines, financial pressure, exams, overwork, and understimulation

- *social factors*: relationship disputes, bullying, isolation, family problems, divorce, and death of a loved one

We also distinguish between acute and chronic stress triggers. *Acute* stress triggers, such as a work deadline or a single exam, are temporary. *Chronic* stressors — such as nursing a sick relative, financial difficulties, taking care of a disabled child, a conflict-filled job situation, or ongoing relationship problems — put a strain on us over a longer period of time. There are also foreseeable stressors (such as a job interview, a wedding, preparing an income tax return) and unforeseeable stressors (such as an accident or getting laid off from a job).

Take a moment to jot down your own typical stress triggers. Identifying our own stressors is an important step in reducing or shifting the negative effect they can have on us.

The Stress Reaction

The human body's reaction to a stressor is a highly complex process. It involves a rapid information transfer through the nervous system and a subsequent surge and release of different so-called stress hormones, including adrenaline, noradrenaline, and cortisol. If the stress reaction continues, other hormones, such as serotonin, dopamine, and the body's own endorphins, will also be released. The stress response has an adaptive function as well as a protective one. This is what makes stress so useful — it provides us with the energy required to take quick action when meeting life's challenges. As Dr. Selye puts it, "Stress is the spice of life."

The stress reaction is a highly active state that is also known as hyperarousal or the fight-or-flight response (so called because the body, on a physiological level, is reacting to danger by preparing to either fight or flee). The hormone cortisol is released, which makes our body — especially our organs and muscles — ready for activity. A healthy person's cortisol level will be highest in the morning, offering more energy at the beginning of daily activities.

The stress reaction takes place automatically and simultaneously on a number of different levels:

- *Physiological*: an adaptive reaction is set in motion, involving increased release of the stress hormones and the body's entrance into fight-or-flight mode. The effects include raised blood pressure, accelerated heartbeat, heightened muscle tension, and reduced digestive activity.
- *Mental*: the mind races, often full of anxiety-provoking thoughts, including negative thinking like: "I can't do this." Conversely, the mind may go blank or become panicked.
- *Emotional*: we may experience helplessness, anger, or anxiety as well as inner restlessness, which can paralyze us and augment the stress. There may also be a feeling of euphoria as a result of increased activity and the adrenaline release.
- *Behavioral*: this category includes diverse effects, including overeating or not eating at all, smoking, increased caffeine consumption, talking fast, hyperactivity, and substance abuse.

Certain reactions can exacerbate the manifestation of stress. For example, when we are frightened and experience a dry mouth and racing heart, this can increase whatever fear is present. If fear increases, it will affect our thinking, turning it to negative or panicked thoughts. It may even lead to thoughts of doom, such as: "I can't take this anymore" or "I wish I could die" or "I think I'm going crazy." At this point we are in danger of getting caught in a downward-spiral stress cycle fed by negative thoughts, which in turn leads to more feelings of fear, anger, or helplessness. In this way the negative thoughts are again reinforced. Simultaneously these emotions, combined with disturbing thoughts, cause a hormonal imbalance in our bloodstream and, in the long term, affect our immune system and heart.

Mindful awareness of our stress triggers and reactions can diminish or alleviate the harmful elements of the stress reaction. Through careful observation of our reactions, we can become more aware of our thoughts and emotions. This in turn makes it easier to avoid being overwhelmed by them. As noted earlier, we can learn to observe our thoughts as "mental events" without getting caught up in their content. As we do this, we strengthen our capacity to note which thoughts are worthy of pursuit, rather than allowing them to govern us.

A Positive Challenge for One Person May Be a Stress Trigger for Another

Stress research has made many advances over the decades, progressing from a mechanistic view to a model that embraces the dynamic relationship between people and their environment. Although stress research still works on the assumption that a stress response follows a stressor, we also know that what constitutes a negative stress trigger for one person may be a welcome challenge or just routine for someone else. For me (Petra), giving lectures used to be a huge source of stress. At the beginning of my career, I had little experience with giving talks. I saw lecturing as a difficult and daunting task. I even turned down some requests to give lectures because I felt I couldn't do it. I worked on my personal assessment of stress triggers and began to practice MBSR, and today I rise to the challenge and enjoy giving talks.

This is a good illustration of what the American psychologist Richard Lazarus meant when he created the transactional model of stress: our experience of stress and the effect of a stressor on our well-being depend largely on our perception of it. This in turn is influenced by how we evaluate our capacity to cope with the stress situation.

Therein lie both the good news and the bad. Based on Lazarus's theory, we can do something to minimize our perceived stress and reduce our reactions — namely, we can be mindful of our mental processes when we are faced with a potential stress trigger. This also gives us the means to take more responsibility for our health and the way we live.

If the causes of our stress were entirely external, we would be at the mercy of our surroundings. This is not the case! Even in the most difficult circumstances, we can learn to maintain our equilibrium and considerably ease our stress levels. There are impressive examples of this, such as Nelson Mandela, who spent decades in prison but never lost his spirit, and Tibetan monks and nuns who are tortured yet who express compassion for their tormentors. Although these are extreme examples, they serve to illustrate the principle that even in the most adverse circumstances we can choose our mind-set as we process and cope with difficult experiences.

Should We Just Grin and Bear It?

Please don't misunderstand us — we don't mean that mindfulness practice dooms us to passively observing and enduring difficult situations and adverse circumstances. On the contrary, mindfulness can lead us to be more clearly aware of unfair or disagreeable conditions in our private and work lives, and then we can decide on the best course of action to remedy them. This might include asking for a raise, changing jobs, having a talk to clear the air, or ending a relationship.

The way we respond to stress is a highly complex, automatic, and conditioned process, one that helps our bodies to adapt to life's changing realities. As a result, the stress response has a protective function. The extent to which we experience a potential stress trigger as a threat — and consequently as a stress factor — determines in no small part (or entirely, according to some researchers) our subsequent assessment of this stressor, whether consciously or unconsciously. Our attitudes, skills, and capabilities — that is, our tools for tackling difficulties — are crucial to how we respond to and handle stress. If we deem the situation manageable and our resources sufficient to come to meet the challenge, our stress response will be markedly lower and briefer than if we assume we're not able to cope with the situation.

This is where stress-amplifying thoughts play an important role — they tend to occur automatically (that is, subconsciously) and result in our viewing something or someone as a stress trigger, which causes us to shift into stress response mode. Typical stress-amplifying thoughts include:

"I'll never manage that."
"I'm not good enough at this."
"I would rather do it myself."
"I want to please everyone."
"I've got to get everything right, all the time."

Stress-amplifying thoughts are associated with our inner demands and the resultant behavior and with feelings. Classic amplifiers of stress thoughts include perfectionism, fear of failure or making mistakes, fear of rejection, the desire to have everything under control, and excessive fear of helplessness.

Stress is not a linear, mechanistic process (if A happens, then B will be the result) but rather a highly individualistic matter. A stress trigger for one person may not be one for another. And because the experience of stress and the resultant effects on our health are so personal and, at the same time, largely subconscious or unconscious, it is important for us to be aware of what takes place on the physiological, mental, emotional, and behavioral levels during a stressful situation. As far as we are concerned, nothing is better suited to training people to become aware of these factors than the practice of mindfulness.

At this point, we would like to introduce an exercise that helps cultivate awareness in everyday life. Practiced regularly, it can help you interrupt the stress cycle. Psychologists John Teasdale, Zindel Segal, and Mark Williams developed this exercise as part of their Mindfulness-Based Cognitive Therapy program.[15] Since it takes only three to five minutes, you may find it easy to fit into your daily routine.

Exercise: Taking Time for a Breathing Space

- Start by sitting in a comfortable, upright position, in a posture that expresses for you an attitude of presence and alertness, dignity, and openness. You may close your eyes or, if you prefer, keep your eyes open but focused downward in a soft gaze.

- Begin by asking yourself: "What is going on in my mind and in my body right now?" Don't try to change anything, but open your awareness to what is present in your body and mind at this moment. It may help to ask yourself: "What thoughts are running through my mind? What emotions am I feeling? What physical sensations?" Notice as gently as you can.

- In the second step, turn your attention to the sensations you experience as you breathe, allowing your awareness to settle in a part of the body where you sense the breath clearly. Be aware as best you can of the breath for the full duration of each inhalation and exhalation, as well as in the pause between breaths.

- In the third step, expand your field of awareness from your breath to your whole body. Sense both the entire space that your physical body takes up and any sensations that may be manifesting in your body at this moment. Observe them in a spirit of kindness, as if your whole body is breathing. If you have particularly intense sensations, see if you can be aware of them as they are, without trying to change them in any way. If you wish, you may experiment with letting the breath flow to these body parts as you breathe in and, possibly, softening as you breathe out.

- Bring the exercise to a close at your own pace.

In the first step of the breathing-space exercise, we take time to focus our attention on the present moment. The exercise invites us to step out of the usual goal-oriented mode of consciousness and instead connect with what we are observing and encountering in the here and now, without judging or trying to change it. You might become aware of thoughts you don't particularly like, or encounter tension in some parts of the body. This phase of the exercise is not about doing anything with the experience, but about acknowledging that it is there. Tell yourself: "It's okay for me to have this thought. I am allowed to feel this way. It's okay that I'm tense." This may provide great relief.

In the second step, we practice becoming aware of our inhalations and exhalations. This usually helps steady the breath, improving our ability to focus on the present, even if our thoughts have a tendency to wander. For a few moments we allow ourselves to interrupt the stream of constant busyness and ride the waves of the breath — the inhaling, exhaling, and pauses in between — as well as the sensations we experience while doing the exercise.

The third step of the exercise can help us broaden our perspective, experience mental relaxation, and return to our daily tasks with a new, fresh vigor. At this stage we let our awareness shift from observing our thoughts to experiencing awareness of our whole body. In doing so, we may sense an inner as well as an outer spaciousness that helps us observe things from a wider perspective.

This exercise is most effective if you practice it regularly. For two weeks try doing the breathing-space exercise first thing after getting home from work or school each day. Or you may prefer to do the exercise in the morning before you leave the house or when you first get to the office, before you turn on your computer. Experiment with finding ways to include the breathing space in your daily life and observe what difference, if any, it makes for you.

Angelika, who works in a hospital, described the effects of the breathing-space exercise as follows:

Whenever I notice that the stress on the ward is getting the better of me — in other words, when I start running around like a
chicken without a head, forgetting things and repeatedly thinking,
"I just can't cope with all this! How on earth is it all supposed to
get done in a day's work?" — I remember the breathing exercise. I go to the restroom for a few minutes, where I can practice
without being disturbed. After that, when I return to the ward, I
see the situation differently. I am more relaxed and able to do one
thing at a time. Situations run more smoothly, and I manage to do
all the things I thought were too difficult to accomplish before.
And even if there's something I don't get around to, I'm able to
remain calm knowing that it can wait until tomorrow.

When Stress Becomes a Habit

There is another reason why stress is such a problem in modern society
and why so many people regularly suffer from its effects. The stress
response puts the body on alert and initiates the fight-or-flight reaction we described earlier — a highly charged state. Every one of our
sinews is programmed to spring into action for the purpose of fighting
or fleeing. This is a primal reaction, one that was helpful in the distant
past when we were struggling for survival, but it is rarely necessary
today. In fact, such a reaction would be completely inappropriate in
most situations. As a rule, modern stress factors are less threatening to
life and limb but nevertheless have a strong effect on our self-esteem
and social status, or on our need for respect, acceptance, attention, and
love. When we deny difficulties and avoid facing our fears, we're taking flight from seemingly desperate situations on a psychological level.

Social or emotional stressors trigger exactly the same fight-or-flight
response as actual physical or threatening situations do. What happens
to the physical preparation the body has experienced (increased muscle tension, etc.) when fight or flight does not occur? The stress reaction turns inward: we internalize it in our bodies. If we do not find a
way to relieve this acute stress, it can become chronic and have serious

consequences for our health, including ongoing tension, cardiovascular problems, elevated blood pressure, internal agitation, low mood, anxiety, or depression.

Stress is part of our daily reality. Because we often have no healthy outlet for this energy and the accompanying feelings, the hormones remain in our bloodstreams rather than being absorbed as they would in the fight-or-flight response. As discussed earlier, this state of keeping the stress response bottled up (instead of fighting or fleeing) is reinforced — and to some extent expected — by our society. Behaviors such as understanding our feelings, recognizing our weaknesses, and taking adequate rest periods — which would help us deal with stress — are given little support in our society, especially in the workplace and in educational settings.

When Work Is the Most Important Thing in Life

People who enjoy their jobs and see them as a way of enhancing their self-esteem and sense of accomplishment may throw themselves into work to the point of getting lost in it. This situation, described in detail by psychologists Zindel V. Segal, J. Mark G. Williams, and John D. Teasdale in their book *Mindfulness-Based Cognitive Therapy for Depression* (2002, 2012), has also been explored by Professor Marie Asberg of the Karolinska Institutet in Stockholm. She demonstrated that when our lives are stressful, we tend to stop doing the things that would normally alleviate that stress.

For example, we might stop going to the movies, meeting friends, or spending time on hobbies. Consequently, our lives become increasingly narrow, until all that's left is work or the other stress factors that are robbing us of energy and motivation. At the same time, we can develop symptoms such as despondency, listlessness, guilt, sleeping disorders, mood swings, and even depression. What's more, Professor Asberg discovered that those most affected by this diminished quality of life are the people who are most conscientious and committed to work and whose sense of self depends primarily on their career success

— in other words, those who are regarded as efficient and accomplished in our society. Asberg's research demonstrates that it's not just unemployment and on-the-job tension that can have adverse effects on our health. A successful career and the initial contentment that comes with it can be just as damaging if we are not mindful and do not counterbalance the strains it can exert.

If we wait for chronic stress symptoms — sleep disorders, high blood pressure, lethargy, memory loss, digestive problems, susceptibility to infections, or even a heart attack — to manifest, our bodies may already be weakened so much that it could take many weeks, months, or even years to recuperate, if we do so at all.

Frequently, a physical or emotional collapse is preceded by harmful "coping" strategies, including excessive consumption of addictive substances such as coffee, alcohol, cigarettes, or even prescription drugs, all of which initially have a soothing effect but are ultimately destructive once addiction kicks in. Helpful stress management calls for strategies and habits that support us in dealing with short-term pressures and strains without allowing them to become chronic stressors that make us ill. At the same time, we must give priority to developing a way of life that enables us to be in touch with our needs and ourselves in a mindful manner, ensuring the delicate balance between tension and relaxation.

How Mindfulness Can Help with Stress

We can reduce stress through mindfulness by learning to recognize stressors and the stress reaction. This involves taking a mindful pause during activity so that we can make conscious decisions.

When we invite mindfulness into normally automatic processes, that action in itself is wholesome because it helps us widen our perception. In other words, the moment we notice we are not being mindful, we are in fact practicing mindfulness.

We can apply this principle to our experience of stress. When a person says, "I am stressed," and pauses to become aware of the bodily sensation of breathing, he or she has already ended an automatic reaction and taken the first step toward responding to the situation in a different way. Once we have learned and practiced mindfulness, we can develop the ability to observe and reflect in a mindful way. Awareness and nonjudgmental observation help create mental and emotional space for actions, and this can lead to adopting more helpful ways of coping with a situation or problem. That way, decisions do not arise from automatic-pilot mode — subconscious, habitual patterns — and the response is creative rather than automatic.

One example of making a conscious choice to mitigate a stress reaction came from Kathrin in the third session of an MBSR course. She told us she had come to realize that she automatically turned on the radio the minute she got into her car, and that it wasn't always good for her. She had done this for years without giving it a second thought.

> Last week I got into the car and switched on the radio without being consciously aware of doing it. I'd had a tough day at the office, and I was emotionally drained and tired. I was worrying about the shopping I still had to do and a parents' association meeting and whether my husband would attend or I'd have to go. At the same time, I was thinking about my mother's birthday present, which I still had to buy. All of a sudden I felt an unpleasant pressure in my stomach, followed by heartburn, and I noticed I was drumming nervously on the steering wheel. When I had to stop at a traffic light, I felt a surge of rage.
>
> This brought me to my senses: I remembered my mindfulness course and what I had learned there. I pulled myself together and consciously focused my attention on my breath. Quietly, I thanked the red light that had forced me to stop — and to pause and think. And as I was reflecting and asking myself, "Where is my awareness now; what sensations am I feeling in my body right now?" I realized that I didn't actually like the music that was playing in the background. I wasn't in the mood for more input; what I needed was peace and quiet — this was really clear to me in that moment of mindfulness.
>
> When I turned off the radio, I immediately felt different. I

took a few deep breaths and continued on my way, calmer and more relaxed.

Since then, Kathrin told us, she no longer simply switches on the radio while "on automatic pilot," but turns it on only when she really wants to listen to it, which is far less often than she used to believe. When she does turn it on, she consciously enjoys the music or program that is playing. This illustrates what we mean by "making a conscious choice."

Our example might give the impression that mindfulness is just another technique for coping with stressful situations: you need only be "a bit more mindful," and then everything will work out better. That is not at all what mindfulness is. In fact, if mindfulness is practiced on a regular basis, it has the potential to fundamentally transform the quality of our day-to-day lives.

Stress, the Stress Reaction, and Stress Symptoms

- Stress is a dynamic event whose effects on an individual differ considerably.
- A distinction must be made between stress triggers (stressors) and a stress reaction.
- The stress reaction occurs on four levels: physiological, emotional, mental, and behavioral.
- Coping well with stress through activation of the stress response calls for addressing stress at all levels: physiological, emotional, mental, and behavioral.
- The physiological stress reaction — fight or flight — is an evolutionary response automatically triggered by a stressor.
- The intensity of the stress reaction depends largely on our assessment of the stressor — whether conscious or subconscious — and our stress-amplifying thoughts.

- The abilities and resources we attribute to ourselves in coping with stress play an equally important role in how stress affects us.
- Denial and repression are not helpful in this respect.
- Denial and repression do not reduce the stress reaction. Instead, they often lead to a situation of chronic stress.

Coping with Stress: The Stress Response

- An effective stress response requires a balance between activity and relaxation, meaning both physical relaxation (e.g., exercise) and mental (e.g., meditation).
- At the same time, it is important to be aware of our stress-amplifying thoughts and the accompanying feelings, to find a way out of the stress spiral. This is where mindfulness can help.
- By practicing mindfulness, we can create space between a stress trigger and a stress reaction as we interrupt the process of going on automatic pilot and losing contact with the present moment. This allows for a conscious and wise choice rather than an unconscious, automatic reaction.

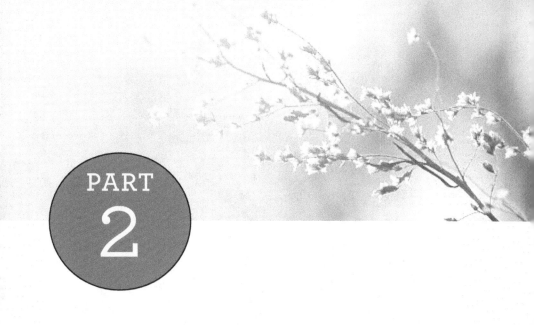

PART 2

The Eight-Week MBSR Course

4 Beginning the Journey: The Mindfulness Compass

B efore we explore the MBSR course week by week, we would like to present some attitudes that we believe are a fundamental part of mindfulness practice. These attitudes are essential qualities that help us practice mindful living and that can enrich our lives significantly. Each of them offers a field of exploration that will invite us, sometimes with urgency, to open, deepen, stretch, and grow.

When we travel somewhere we've never been before, many of us buy guidebooks and study them carefully. One section of a guidebook that is especially helpful explains the customs of the place we plan to visit. For example, in parts of southern Europe, stores close in the afternoon for a long siesta, and dinner is usually eaten at 9 PM or even later. Such information helps us adjust to new cultures and minimize inconveniences. Yet there is a great difference between knowing about and actually experiencing a new place. Being forewarned does not mean we won't encounter difficulties. For example, even though you know that the stores close between noon and 4 PM, you might still get annoyed if you have a bad headache at 12:30 and can't buy a pain reliever because the pharmacy is closed.

Signing up for an MBSR course is like planning a trip, and to help you navigate the journey we would like to introduce what we call the mindfulness compass. The points on our compass correspond to attitudes or perspectives that can support you, and even challenge you, when you take up the practice of MBSR. At any time during the course, you may find yourself moving in the direction of one of these compass points.

MBSR is in fact a journey of coming home to ourselves. Think about those proverbial stories told in many different ways — such as *The Wizard of Oz* — about people who travel to a distant place in search of something, only to return home and discover they had it all along. Coming home in MBSR means to arrive in the present moment, the treasure we were seeking. The present moment is the only one in which we can take action and make choices. We can reflect mindfully on either the past or the future when necessary, without losing ourselves in either one.

The present moment is a time of abundance. While it may be filled with ease, challenge, or both, whether it is pleasant or unpleasant there is a sense of aliveness and a potential for informed choice. How we meet and dwell in each second...each breath...and how we meet and dwell in our lives, is the essence of the mindfulness journey.

It's Not Easy

Anyone who has tried to change a habit knows it can't be done on a whim. The more ingrained the habit, the harder it is to work with. It takes effort, perseverance, and attention to shift or change. *It's not easy.*

The phrase *It's not easy* has become almost taboo in our culture. Programs for personal development, weight loss, anger management, success in business or parenting, and the like often try to mask the truth that it takes motivation, dedication, and commitment to grow, change, or improve. If a self-help book is an honest one, it should include plenty of words like *effort*, *time*, and *perseverance* — and not just in the fine print!

Participation in an MBSR course asks that we practice at home each day for up to one hour with CDs of the formal exercises, such as yoga, the body scan, or the sitting meditation, as well as engage in informal exercises or sometimes in completing a journal entry about a particular theme. A question that many prospective participants ask is: "But what if something happens at work, or whatever, and I can't practice that day?" This is a reasonable thing to ask, but often in asking such a question, we are already looking for the exit before we have entered the room. We've checked out before we have checked in.

No one can know the future. No one can say what will come up during the week that might prevent us from practicing at home. At the same time, mindfulness practice encourages us to reflect and be in touch with the various emotions and/or thoughts that come up, and to be in contact as best we can with our motivations. But rather than assign blame, we reflect kindly and also clearly on what may be arising and work with it as openly as we can. In class we talk about how to keep the practice going even if we can't do it formally, and we are encouraged to examine as best we can how we may either sabotage or discourage our own practice through reacting with harshness if we "slip."

Lively and sometimes difficult exchanges can happen in class in response to the theme of practice. At the same time, the climate is one of reflection and commitment to working with what comes up. We also emphasize that in situations where formal practice is not possible, informal practice, which is also vital, helps us continue to practice mindfulness with integrity.

It's easy to make statements about how much we want to change or gain insight into a behavior. And it's not easy to stay committed and on track, because we are met by all sorts of circumstances and challenges. What is clear, however, is that the more we commit to being with our experience and whatever is coming up, the theme of "it's not easy" loses its relevance and we just practice.

Willingness

During a preinterview for an MBSR course, Robert admitted, "I just don't know if I have the kind of discipline necessary to keep up with the program."

I (Linda) asked, "Can you say what you mean by *discipline*?"

Robert looked at me sideways, raised an eyebrow, and replied, "Well, it's obvious, isn't it? I don't know if I can stick with it. I'm afraid that when the alarm clock rings, I'll do what I always do and roll over and go back to sleep."

"This course has nothing to do with discipline," I said as a gentle challenge.

"Then why all this talk about practicing at home every day and being mindful in daily life?" Robert exclaimed. "Sounds to me like I have to do something all the time. That's work, and work takes discipline."

We explored together how the word *discipline* is often associated with an iron will and the ability to direct ourselves, even force ourselves, to carry out a task. I suggested that the word *willingness* was a more fruitful way to think of what *discipline* could mean in this context. Willingness is an attitude that supports us in practicing mindfulness. It is a readiness to turn toward rather than turn away from a difficult situation. It includes a commitment to trying to be aware of what we are doing when we are doing it. Charlotte Joko Beck, a well-known Zen meditation teacher, writes in *Everyday Zen*: "Discipline has a connotation for some of us of forcing ourselves to do something. But discipline is simply bringing all the light we can summon to bear on our practice, so that we can see a little bit more."[16]

Awakening the spirit of willingness is an important step toward taking conscious action rather than reacting. In order to do something in a different way, we first have to be aware of *what* we are doing. Only then can we get in touch with all the nuances of a situation — sensations, thoughts, emotions — that are present, without trying to either suppress or change them.

Observing — being in contact with all the thoughts and emotions that arise when we're in a situation — is a key element of mindfulness. Before we can change a behavior, we need to be aware of what we are doing. When we are willing to observe ourselves, we can learn a great deal in the process. Take, for example, Robert's experience of not wanting to get up when the alarm rings. He would ignore the alarm clock and turn over to go back to sleep. Many of us might do the same thing. Being mindful, we can notice that we might have a reason for not wanting to get up. Maybe we had to work late or were ill the night before, or we overate and fell into bed completely stuffed, which kept us from sleeping well.

Next, we pay attention to our thoughts. A thought that might arise could be: "Maybe I made a mistake in planning to practice this morning. It's Sunday, after all, and this is normally a day off. Isn't it?"

The attitude that supports willingness is the conscious decision to stay present in the situation rather than to disengage and allow everything to run on as if the brakes are broken. In this case, we may indeed roll over and go back to sleep; but if we are fully in touch with our decision, it is not an unconscious reaction but an aware choice. That is a gift that practicing willingness can give us.

Just Keep Going

In the proverbial story about someone looking for a treasure everywhere and then discovering it in her or his backyard, the hardships of the journey — crossing mountains, fording rivers, and walking over stony territory — play an important role. Think about Dorothy in *The Wizard of Oz* and all the obstacles she faces before she discovers that "there's no place like home." Throughout the journey, the traveler, like Dorothy, keeps going, even though each challenge provides a strong reason to turn back.

There may be times in an MBSR course when you wonder why you embarked on the journey in the first place. It may seem that you are not getting anywhere or that the obstacles are too daunting. It may also feel as if you are going in the wrong direction, or even backward. At that point, it is completely understandable if you shake your compass to see if it's working, or you think about canceling the trip and taking the first plane home.

During the interview or orientation meeting that precedes the MBSR course, we remind participants that making the decision to do the whole eight weeks is their own. When the thought arises that it makes no sense at all to continue, exactly at that moment it's important to recommit. There is power and presence in reminding yourself of your intention to finish the journey you started, not because reaching the goal is the only thing of importance, but because the stops along the way are as much a part of the journey as reaching the end. So if you are stuck, notice the stuckness...and just keep going.

Don't Ask Why...at Least Not Right Now

Asking why is often an important thing to do, yet as far as mindfulness practice is concerned, asking why is like driving down a street that loops back on itself. When we begin, it may seem as if we are going somewhere, but in the end we are just going round and round and round.

We are used to asking, and often encouraged to ask, why. We do it in school, in science, in the courtroom, and in myriad other places. In all of these situations, it is appropriate to pose questions and seek to answer them, but in mindfulness practice we often ask why before we have had a chance to really assess what is going on or understand where we are. Looking for an answer can keep us busy and help create a barrier so that we don't have to experience confusion or the fact that we don't have an answer at all.

In mindfulness practice, why is really not a question. It is a thought that comes up repeatedly that leads to more thinking. It rarely results in a helpful solution to our problems, especially at the early stages of our training.

Does that mean we should never try to find the cause of a situation or a solution to a problem? Of course not, and the fear we will be left adrift without our "why" searchlight often arises.

The most helpful way to work with the question why in the early stages of mindfulness training is to acknowledge it is there but not try to answer it. Notice your tendency to want an explanation, or the feeling of insecurity that prompts the question, and just let it be present without acting on it.

Kindness/Tenderness

At the beginning of our institute's nine-month mindfulness trainings, we ask people to write down their personal goals for the course. We collect the answers and return them at the last meeting. At that point we ask the participants to reflect on how they behaved at the start of the training and where they are now.

The comment expressed in the group most often conveys how hard participants were on themselves when they began the program — how demanding, harsh, cold, and unrelenting they were about the goals they set for themselves. One woman hit the mark when she said, "I would never knowingly choose to treat someone the way I treated myself."

In his book *Meetings at the Edge*, Stephen Levine, a meditation teacher and expert on death and dying, writes, "Kindness to yourself might be the most difficult path you will ever tread, because it is so unexplored and we have so little support for that kind of self mercy."[17]

Kindness toward oneself is a feeling that is foreign to many of our students. Some tell us they have no right to ask it for themselves: kindness is expressed only to someone else. Some identify gentleness toward themselves with weakness: Anything worth having, after all, has to be hard to achieve…doesn't it?

Kindness is a rare gift that we seldom give ourselves. In reality, it is often something we think we have to earn. Kindness for ourselves becomes a commodity that we use to bargain with. For example, we might make ourselves work to the point of exhaustion before allowing ourselves a break.

Perhaps one of the unkindest things we do is try to change ourselves because we think something is wrong with us. We can become fixated on our flaws and even become addicted to the idea of self-improvement. To say, "There is nothing fundamentally wrong with me," sounds like a lie, a brag, or self-delusion. What prevents us from accepting our inherent goodness is a harsh, critical attitude toward ourselves that other people notice but which often goes unnoticed by us.

One of the most destructive applications of this attitude is to tell others (or ourselves) that there is something wrong with them as a way to motivate change. Most research on optimism and on motivation behavior, such as the work of positive psychologist Martin Seligman, shows time and again that we flourish with praise and kind words, and that harsh, unfair, and personally motivated criticism is a form of emotional violence, especially when we internalize it and become our own biggest critic.

Many MBSR course participants say that the cultivation of friendliness toward themselves and the opportunity to experience it is one of the most important aspects of the course. That kindness, which allows them to open their hearts to themselves, helps nurture a new perspective.

During the course, we sometimes present a guided meditation on being kind to ourselves. The responses of course participants can be deeply moving. Once the meditation is over, there is softness in the room — gentleness — and often tears flow. Linda frequently reads a quote from Pema Chödrön, a widely respected American nun in the Tibetan tradition and meditation teacher, who wrote in *The Wisdom of No Escape*: "Meditation practice isn't about trying to throw ourselves away and become something better. It's about befriending who we are already." Many in the group nod in agreement with these wise words that teach kindness and tenderness toward ourselves. We explore this theme in all of its aspects as we progress through the program.

Not Resisting Resistance

One thing that comes up for a number of people in an MBSR course is a sense of resistance. Participants express it in different ways: by not coming to class, not doing a home practice assignment, deliberately ignoring the instructions, criticizing the program, or asking questions that come from a place of rebellion rather than a need to know.

Resistance can feel very convincing. All sorts of counterarguments can sound logical. Yet if we listen closely, we hear the fear underneath the words. Resistance often comes up because we are afraid of change. It may be related to something at work, in our personal relationships, or even in connection to ourselves.

Meeting resistance rather than acting on it does not mean we should deny the need to take action against injustice, abuse, or any kind of destructive behavior. Rather, within the context of mindfulness, we are referring to the kind of resistance that arises when we feel an urge to pull the emergency brake when we are moving in an unfamiliar but not necessarily dangerous direction.

Resistance consumes a great deal of our mental and emotional energy. Like a security guard stationed at an entrance with strict orders not to let anyone in or out, resistance can create an emotional stalemate, not allowing anything to shift in any direction.

The practice of applying mindfulness to resistance is simply this: Be with it. We don't try to get rid of it, change it, inform it, or suppress it. We simply do not feed it. We let it be. We carry our resistance in the most careful and tender way possible and allow it to be present among all the other aspects of our lives.

No matter how resistance manifests, it is usually about saying no to the present moment. And in suggesting how to be with resistance, I (Linda) would say it is not unlike the way we might deal with a child who is going through the "terrible twos," a stage when no matter what is suggested, a two-year-old child is very likely to say, "No!" Imagine that you need to go in one direction and your child is intent on going in another. It does not help to shout no in response to a child's no or to argue with her. It's more helpful to say something like: "I understand you want to go to the playground, but we have to get to the supermarket before it closes." Then take her gently but firmly by the hand, leading her in the direction you need to go, not dragging her but firmly and gently moving forward.

Resistance is an emotional reaction that is part of mindfulness practice. Giving it space and allowing ourselves to be present to our own resistance is a powerful and illuminating exercise. We do not need to resist resistance. Cultivating a gracious step toward it can help us stay present and receive whatever we can learn about ourselves that will help us live a mindful life.

Expectations

There is one certain truth about expectations: everyone has them! When we come to an MBSR class, we expect to learn how mindfulness can help us cope with the stress in our lives. We expect the teacher to be supportive of our process. We expect to apply the lessons to our lives.

Based on the description of the program, these are reasonable things to expect. Equally reasonable is the understanding that changes rarely take place instantly or without some effort on our part. The question becomes: Can we balance our expectations with a dose of reality and respect for the way things are?

Expectations are tricky things. They may seem reasonable, but they turn very quickly into wishes, hopes, and fantasies...and we want all of them met. The sooner the better! Indeed, they can rapidly become longings, even cravings to which we become attached. These can control our behavior and lives, and much of what we do may be focused on satisfying them.

Mary, who suffered from pain in her left knee and was facing yet another operation, had this to say about her expectations: "When I started the MBSR program, it was with a strong expectation that my pain would get better. Or at least, it wouldn't bother me as much. As the fourth week rolled around, I was quite disturbed. It wasn't happening the way it was supposed to." She paused for a moment and then continued:

> If it was only about getting rid of the pain, I would have to say that my expectations have not been satisfied. But other things have happened that I never expected. I actually go out and do things I would not have done before. And I take the time to notice how beautiful the flowers in my garden are. I like to sit there in the

evening and count the stars. Before, I was so wrapped up in my pain, I missed the rest of my life.

Mary's comments point to one of the most harmful aspects of insisting that our expectations be met: we exclude things from our lives that don't match those expectations.

In mindfulness practice, we learn that becoming aware, and even intimate, with our expectations is the most helpful way to soften their controlling effects. Seeing expectations for what they are, in as gentle and friendly a way as possible, can allow us to honor our hopes and, at the same time, ground them in realistic terms.

This does not mean developing an attitude of resignation, or giving up on something or someone, or not taking care of ourselves as best we can. One gift of mindfulness practice is the acceptance that expectations can be the road to true compassion for ourselves. We can honor our humanity and our hopeful wishes, and stay grounded in the fact that we cannot control our lives or circumstances. No matter what our expectations, to some extent what will be will be; and we can do our best to be with that reality as mindfully, kindly, and vitally as we can.

It's Okay to Be Imperfect

Not only is it okay not to be perfect, but it's also, for many participants in MBSR courses, an immense relief to hear this. Why?

The urge for perfection has resulted in incredible works of art and inspiration, but it has also created a myth of excellence that has become the hell of modern life. We long for perfect relationships, perfect homes, perfect cars, perfect jobs, and perfect lives. Everything is compared to an ideal and invariably comes up short because life is not perfect. Life shifts and changes; nothing can remain the same forever. It is messy, dirty, and full of mishaps, as well as straight, squeaky clean, and perfectly ordered. It can be exquisitely beautiful and painfully ugly and everything in between.

In mindfulness practice you may hear: "As it is, it is perfect" or

"It's *okay*." That might sound confusing at first, like a contradiction of what I said in the previous paragraph, but *perfect* or *okay* in this instance refers to the sense that each thing is unique, each person is unique, and that rather than strive for a perfection that does not exist, we can honor the integrity of something exactly as it is.

One day a student in an MBSR course brought in the following article. She handed it to me with the words "It's okay not to be perfect."

The Broken Violin

The following article appeared in the *Houston Chronicle* on February 10, 2001. However, there is some doubt as to whether the event really occurred. Whatever its veracity, the story has circulated as part of a tradition of folklore known as urban legends — stories that take hold of the popular imagination and often go viral, but which in fact probably never happened.[18]

On November 18, 1995, Itzhak Perlman, the violinist, came on stage to give a concert at Avery Fisher Hall at Lincoln Center in New York City. If you have ever been to a Perlman concert, you know that getting on stage is no small achievement for him. He was stricken with polio as a child, and so he has braces on both legs and walks with the aid of two crutches. To see him walk across the stage one step at a time, painfully and slowly, is an unforgettable sight. He walks painfully, yet majestically, until he reaches his chair. Then he sits down, slowly, puts his crutches on the floor, undoes the clasps on his legs, tucks one foot back and extends the other foot forward. Then he bends down and picks up the violin, puts it under his chin, nods to the conductor and proceeds to play.

By now, the audience is used to this ritual. They sit quietly while he makes his way across the stage to his chair. They remain reverently silent while he undoes the clasps on his legs. They wait until he is ready to play.

But this time, something went wrong. Just as he finished the first few bars, one of the strings on his violin broke. You could hear it snap — it went off like gunfire across the room. There was no mistaking what that sound meant. There was no mistaking what he had to do.

People who were there that night thought to themselves: "We figured that he would have to get up, put on the clasps again, pick up the crutches and limp his way off stage — to either find another violin or else find another string for this one."

But he didn't. Instead, he waited a moment, closed his eyes and then signaled the conductor to begin again. The orchestra began, and he played from where he had left off. And he played with such passion and such power and such purity as they had never heard before.

Of course, anyone knows that it is impossible to play a symphonic work with just three strings. I know that, and you know that, but that night, Itzhak Perlman refused to know that.

Non-Doing

Perhaps one of the most elusive aspects of mindfulness practice is doing without doing — what we call non-doing. "That's a contradiction," class participants often say. "If I want something to happen, I have to do something."

This is true. However, non-doing, or effortless effort, is really about how we accomplish tasks and how we live our lives.

I (Linda) recently read a story in a magazine about how parents push their children at younger and younger ages to study foreign languages, solve math problems, and excel at playing musical instruments. One of the illustrations for the article showed a puzzle with round, square, and triangular holes. Next to it were broken pieces in the same shapes...and a hammer. The implication was that someone had tried to force the pieces to go where they didn't belong.

In our modern lives, we have become addicted to effort. It seems normal to strive to go faster and higher and to achieve more of everything. At the same time, the effects of such a lifestyle show up in the number of people suffering from physiological and psychological stress-related conditions. These ailments are developing at an alarming rate throughout the entire population, particularly among children and youth.

The phrase *effortless effort* seems to presents a paradox or contradiction. One of the gifts of paradox, however, is that it invites us not to take things at face value, to instead question and look more closely. It gives us the opportunity to ask, "What could effortless effort mean for me in terms of the way I live my life?" This leads naturally to another question: "What kind of effort is stressful?"

And indeed, it becomes clear for many MBSR course participants that it is not the activity itself but all the extra elements that we attach to it that creates stress: the merciless drive to get it right, the fear of making a mistake, the going beyond our own physical limits. Instead of allowing a natural unfolding, we push and push, maintaining a blind faith that "just a bit more" is a good thing.

Nature is a master of effortless effort. Flowers bloom, snow falls, and the seasons come and go, yet there are many ways human beings try to force nature, often with disastrous consequences. An example of this is a story quoted in the book *Zorba the Greek* by Nikos Kazantzakis about a young boy who observes a butterfly in its cocoon. Seeing the insect struggling to get out, he takes pity on it and cuts the cocoon open to release the insect. The butterfly emerges, lives for a few moments, and then collapses and dies.

The butterfly was simply not yet ready to leave the cocoon. Mother Nature designed this process wisely: The very effort that a butterfly normally makes to get out of the cocoon is what helps its wings fill with fluid and grow strong. Releasing it early interferes with this natural process of metamorphosis.

The practice of effortless effort will not only have a deep effect on your meditation practice but will also spread through your life in a way that allows you to "just be." Rather than emulating the young boy who did not let the butterfly emerge naturally, we can experience the healing quality of just being, just allowing life to unfold as we bear witness with our bodies, minds, and hearts.

5 The Eight-Week MBSR Program

essions of the eight-week MBSR course take place once a week and generally last two and a half to three hours. The course also includes an all-day retreat (what we call the Day of Mindfulness) that usually takes place between the sixth and seventh classes.

Before taking part in an MBSR course, students are usually invited to an individual interview or an orientation seminar. This gives them the opportunity to get to know the MBSR teacher, familiarize themselves with the course and its requirements, and decide whether they want to take part. The teacher asks about students' health and stress factors and what brought them to consider taking part in an MBSR course. Prospective students also have a chance to ask questions about the program and to explore their goals and discuss whether these are realistic. The teacher explains the importance of the commitment to practice daily at home, and together teacher and student may reflect on how the home practice can be included in daily life. Based on the information they receive, people can decide whether an MBSR course is right for them.

A Short Overview of the MBSR Course Contents

- Each class includes practice in one or more of the formal mindfulness exercises taught in an MBSR course: the body scan, mindful yoga, sitting meditation, or walking meditation.

- After the formal practice, there is time for students to share and further explore their experiences with the exercises conducted during class and their daily practice at home.
- Each class session has a theme (e.g., the meaning of mindfulness, the origins of stress, mindful communication, mindful self-care), which is explored in thematic exercises and in group sharing sessions. The emphasis is on the integration of mindfulness into daily life.
- The participants receive a workbook and CDs for the formal exercises so they can practice at home.
- In addition to the weekly assignments, the workbook includes explanatory material, poems, stories, and further suggestions for integrating mindfulness into everyday life.
- Both the formal exercises and the informal ones, where we engage in daily activity mindfully, are important components of mindfulness practice.

Mindfulness in Everyday Life

When we start practicing mindfulness, we soon notice how restless and distracted we are and how difficult it is to remain focused on something so seemingly simple as, for example, breathing. A small noise is all it takes to flood the mind with associations, memories, and thoughts related to this sound. Before we know it, we are caught up in a story that has nothing to do with our experience in the here and now. Keeping our attention focused on the present requires regular practice and ongoing effort. Wishing alone won't bring it about. There is no better place to practice than in our daily lives. That's why practicing formal meditation exercises, as well as what we call "informal mindfulness practice," on a daily basis is an essential part of every MBSR course.

The informal exercises include going about daily activities — such as climbing the stairs, ironing, washing the dishes, showering, tidying up, cooking, and eating — in a mindful way. Being mindful in this context means being present during the activity — alert and with a sense of genuine curiosity. We do our best to execute these activities with awareness and a mind-set that expresses interest. This means that when we wash the dishes, we wash the dishes, and we also feel the warm water, the dishes, our posture, and ourselves in contact with our breath.

Not everyone is overly enthusiastic at first about being mindful. Some say, "But I don't want to be consciously aware of every second of my life. I'm glad I can wash the dishes now and then without having to think about it. And anyway, it would take far too long doing it this way." Another objection that is often voiced is: "Why would I want to be in contact with things, especially when they are painful or emotionally difficult? Sometimes I just want to escape."

Often these same participants say later in the course that they realized this very attitude caused them to miss parts of their lives. Learning to stay with an experience, even when we feel we want to run away, brings richness and a sense of wholeness that many participants come to value. Over time, this helps us develop inner strength, stability, and resilience, even while the storms of life are raging.

A part of our lives consists of routine activities. In mindfulness practice our daily chores become wake-up bells that remind us we can be present to our lives. Showing up for life is what mindfulness is all about.

Informal mindfulness practice often raises questions such as:

- Am I living this particular moment to the fullest?
- Am I really present in my life?
- Am I stuck in the past or living in the hope of a better future?

At the end of her eight-week course, Elizabeth shared her experiences with practicing mindfulness in daily life:

I feel that every moment in which I mindfully tidy up, wash the dishes, or take care of the children, I am recapturing my life. I have experienced how liberating it is not to see everything as a chore or have the attitude that the actual good, relaxed life only starts when my working day ends. That way I miss out on my whole life, because in the evenings I am tired and put it off till the next day. I practiced for eight weeks to decide for myself what was really important in my daily life, and also to be more aware of the good moments.

If this resonates with you, we suggest that you — just like the participants of an MBSR course, choose a daily activity, such as washing the dishes, showering, climbing the stairs, or brushing your teeth, and be mindful whenever you do it over the course of a week. Notice as best you can how it affects your experience of the activity and whether any lessons you learn spill over into daily life.

Exploring Mindfulness

In the first meeting of an MBSR course, we do something that we rarely do in daily life: we take time to introduce ourselves to one another. We also take time to listen to the stories of why people have come to this class...on this evening...in this place.

As people begin to share information about themselves, the effort that each of them has made to come to class becomes apparent. All have had to find time in their busy lives. Transportation arrangements had to be made. Other people are often involved in helping someone attend the course, by babysitting the kids, filling in at work, looking after a pet.

It is no accident that these participants make such an effort to be in an MBSR class. Their reasons are expressed in different ways, but each one reveals the same impulse: coming to class is an acknowledgment that things cannot go on the way they have been.

For many it's their present situation. It might be an illness or a problem at work or in a relationship. Fear of loss is another strong motivation, whether it pertains to our job or the life of a loved one. Chronic pain, tension in the family, living with a major illness, a sense that life has lost its meaning, a move to a new city, or a divorce can each take a toll. Many people are worn down by the realities of their lives — busyness, confusion, health challenges, work insecurities, loss of community or family connection, and frustrated dreams.

A second theme also becomes apparent as participants listen to each other: signing up for an MBSR class is a step toward doing something for themselves. For many, this is a completely new experience.

What stops so many of us from helping ourselves? When we ask this question, often another one pops up: "Do I have the right to do something only for myself?" For many people, this is a difficult question. For a parent, taking personal time means being away from his or her children. Someone with a demanding job feels it's unfair to leave work early and ask others to cover for her. A son with an aging father worries that something may go wrong while he is away.

For many participants, the idea that it is wrong or selfish to take care of ourselves is rarely questioned. This is an example of how mindfulness can play a revolutionary role in our lives. As we continue to practice, we may well begin to question or reflect on things that we used to take for granted. This can open up a new world of possibilities.

The Class Experience

Many participants in MBSR courses say that being together in a group is one of the most important elements of the course. There is a sense of community and of sharing a common goal: to be more in touch with a life that until now has felt overwhelming.

To support the group process, MBSR teachers usually mention some ground rules that everyone is asked to honor. These include the following:

- All individuals in the group can share as much or as little about themselves as they wish.
- Students respect the privacy of each participant by not talking about any classmates outside of class or mentioning anyone's name.
- Participants are asked to telephone or email the teacher to let him or her know when they cannot attend a class.
- We introduce guidelines for engaging in mindful communication by asking participants:

1. not to interrupt each other.
2. to refrain from offering advice or suggestions.
3. to speak from their own experience.
4. to refrain from judging others.

Why do we ask people to refrain from offering advice or telling someone what he or she is doing wrong? Anna expresses how this guideline helped her:

> I have spent most of my life feeling like a ghost... talking to people but no one seeming to listen. In this class, I felt listened to for the first time. And it had nothing to do with the fact of whether someone agreed with me or not. That, in the end, was not important. Being listened to without judgment or someone telling me what I should do made me feel appreciated. I felt seen and heard.

First Mindfulness Practice: The Raisin Exercise

In the raisin exercise (described on pages 18–21), we explored a small dried fruit with the five senses (sight, touch, hearing, smell, and taste), as we do during the first session of an MBSR course. In the class discussions that follow this exercise, certain attitudes that play a prominent role in our lives are pointed out:

- We are quick to judge something in terms of our likes and dislikes.
- Habits are very strong, and we are often unaware of them.
- We miss or ignore a great deal in life because we think we know about something already.
- We don't allow ourselves to be receptive to new experiences.
- Our thoughts are often about the past or the future.

As we ate the raisin, we practiced paying attention to all the phases of the experience. This allowed us to center and anchor ourselves in moment-to-moment reality.

For the rest of the course, indeed the rest of your life, the lessons of the raisin exercise can be with you. One course participant expressed it this way:

> I had packed a bag of raisins in my suitcase to snack on. Somehow the package broke open, and the raisins spilled everywhere. I tried to clean them up the best I could. But for the rest of the trip, I was constantly discovering new raisins each time I pulled out an article of clothing.
>
> I was annoyed and worried that they would stain my clothes. At the same time, I was reminded of the lessons of the raisin that I had learned during the MBSR class: every moment is unique and precious, and I do not want to waste a single one. It was as if a mindfulness bell rang each time I found a slightly squashed raisin.
>
> What a sweet moment!

The Body Scan

After the raisin exercise, we introduce participants to the body scan. The body scan is the first so-called formal exercise that we practice in MBSR. During the body scan we move our awareness through the body from the toes to the head, paying attention to each body part, taking note of what we experience when we place our attention there. In particular, we notice any sensations (such as tingling, itching, pressure), temperature changes, lightness or heaviness, tension or spaciousness. We may also notice nothing in particular when a part of the body is mentioned, and then we are encouraged to simply be aware of "nothing in particular." Rather than look for anything or try to produce something to notice, we rest in an open awareness of whatever arises from moment to moment.

The intent of the body scan is to experience all the different parts of the body with the same mindful attention we applied to the raisin. In a body scan of the left leg, for example, we scan the leg in the following sequence, opening to whatever is present — or not — in that region of the body:

- the toes of the foot
- the big toe
- the small toe
- all the toes in between
- the ball...then we move to the arch
- the heel
- the top of the foot
- the left foot as a whole
- the ankle
- the lower leg
- the calf
- the shinbone
- the knee
- the kneecap
- the back of the knee
- the thigh, bottom, and then the top of the left leg

For the remainder of the exercise we scan the rest of the body in the same detail, moving to the right leg, the buttocks, the pelvis, the upper body, the arms, and the neck and head region, including the face. At the end of the body scan, we practice a full-body breathing exercise and then end with a few minutes of stillness.

Following the body scan, we take time for participants to share their experiences. The first class ends in a review of the home practice and other assignments in the workbook.

Why Do We Practice the Body Scan?

During the body scan, we also introduce a key aspect of mindfulness: paying attention without judgment. In beginning mindfulness practice, one of the first things we see is how often we want things to be different from what they are. We may think we should not be having a particular sensation, or we are not experiencing what we think we should or how we would like it to be. We may drift into random thinking or feeling sleepy (even falling asleep), and as a result we feel we are not doing the body scan correctly. Just how critical of ourselves we can be is surprising — and disturbing — for many students as they begin mindfulness practice.

At the same time, seeing how we so often fall into judging ourselves allows us to begin practicing an important mindfulness skill: noticing, or becoming aware, that we are judging, and then gently letting the judging stop and returning our attention to where we are in the body scan. We may feel a pull to keep going down the road of self-judgment, but with continued mindfulness practice we learn that we can choose to take the road of mindful awareness again and again.

Nothing that we experience in mindfulness training is not part of the practice. Like life, things happen all the time. As John Lennon sung so wisely in the song "Beautiful Boy (Darling Boy)": "Life is what happens to you while you're busy making other plans." That is a given. How we respond, however, is something we can influence.

For example, during the body scan we practice exercising mindful choice. The first step is to become aware that we do indeed have a choice, though we often have to strengthen our mindfulness muscle first, because the tendency to react is so strong. With time we can move from automatic reacting to mindful responding, which means we become aware that we can respond in a different way.

There is something powerful in being part of a group of people lying on the floor practicing the body scan. It is also touching to observe as each member of the class moves to arrange his or her practice space, taking care to make himself or herself comfortable (something we often rush through in daily life). We may sense that, as different as participants are in the class, they share an intention to dive into mindfulness practice and do their very best. What is often a group of very different people becomes a community of people who at least for the moment are willing to explore the possibility of being awake and aware in their own bodies.

Aspects of the Body Scan

- The body scan introduces one of the core principles of mindfulness practice: to be with what is, without trying to change or control the situation.
- The body scan offers the opportunity to practice key aspects of mindfulness, including learning to:
  1. direct our attention in a certain way.
  2. notice when our attention drifts away.
  3. return to the present moment.
  4. be aware of habitual reactions, including judging, rejection, avoidance, and so on.
  5. be aware of our own preferences and prejudices.
  6. become aware of the difference between thinking about something and sensing it with awareness.

- The body scan is a way to get out of the head and back into the body. We are so often out of touch with our physical body and the signals and wisdom it can offer us. We often reject it, try to change it, and push beyond its healthy limits. We take the body for granted and think of it more as a machine than as the embodiment of all that is human in us.
- The body scan invites us to be aware of the entire body, including parts that cause problems, in a new or different way. We are offered the possibility to get to know what we may have pushed away for a long time. In doing so, we may see that the pushing away causes far more pain than coming in contact and being intimate with the very parts we wanted to banish.
- In the body scan, we encourage people to take care of themselves by finding a suitable posture and arranging to have all that they need at their disposal

(blankets, pillows, etc.). The theme of self-care is discussed throughout the course.

- One important aspect of the body scan is also the possibility of experiencing the body as a whole. The feeling of unity can be experienced at any time, even if we are ill or living with pain.

- People coping with pain often come to recognize that they are more than their pain. In the body scan they can also experience parts of their body that are not in pain.

- A body scan is not a relaxation exercise. It is an exercise in mindfulness designed to nurture wakefulness and attentiveness. Participants may not understand this at first, since relaxation is often a strong goal and lying down is usually associated with relaxing or going to sleep.

Helpful Suggestions for Practicing the Body Scan

1. Sometimes participants ask if they can move during a body scan. Such a question is really a lead-in to reflecting on the difference between conscious choice and automatic reaction. We can practice being aware of the impulse to move and, at that moment, choose not to but rather to observe what is coming up. We can also make a decision to move and then do so slowly, being aware so that it becomes mindful movement. In practicing like this, we explore the difference between reaction and response.

2. Some participants associate breathing into and out of a part of the body as a tool to get rid of pain or to relax. We do not use the breath to get rid of anything, including pain, tension, discomfort, and restlessness, when we practice the body scan.

3. The body scan is as much about directing the awareness to a

part of the body as it is about letting go and moving on to the next part. You may find you wish to remain longer in a particular part of the body. At other times you may feel that the guidance of the body scan is too slow. Here it is helpful to see that we can attach ourselves to a particular way of doing things, and that we have strong likes and dislikes.

The following suggestions are based on those in *Mindfulness-Based Cognitive Therapy for Depression.*[19]

1. Whatever experiences you have during the body scan are part of the exercise. These may include falling asleep, forgetting where you are in the meditation, being aware of unpleasant — or pleasant — feelings or sensations, or losing your concentration. As best you can, see if it is possible to be aware of them, just as they are. No need to change anything.

2. Each time your mind wanders, note the thoughts gently (as passing events in the mind), and then bring the mind back to the body scan.

3. There is a tendency to approach such exercises as if they are a competition. It is helpful to notice this (since it gives you insight into a prevalent way we create stress for ourselves). And after noticing, let go of the need to perform well, of any notions about succeeding or failing, of wanting to do the scan properly. Nurturing an attitude of genuine interest, of curiosity, is most helpful in this respect. Then, let the rest take care of itself.

4. Rather than cultivating expectations about and hopes for what the body scan will do for you, imagine instead that you are sowing a seed. The more you poke at a seed and interfere, the less likely it is to grow. The same goes for the body scan. Just keep watering the soil by practicing, and be patient. You never know when a sprout of wisdom will burst through the soil.

The Gift of Mindfulness

The role that mindfulness can play in our lives is introduced in Week 1 of an MBSR course. In the weeks that follow, these aspects will become apparent in all their nuances. Like a crystal held up to the sun and spun to reveal numerous different angles, our lives will unfold in all of their subtlety and variety.

One key aspect that many participants become aware of is the tendency to focus on everything about ourselves and our situation that is *not* okay. On the subject of mindfulness, Jon Kabat-Zinn said, "As long as you are breathing, there is more right with you than wrong with you, no matter what is wrong."

Against this background, an important aspect of the MBSR course can be described like this: Each of us has the resources and abilities to cope with problems in our lives, and they can be strengthened by practicing mindfulness. Learning to cultivate a nonjudgmental attitude helps us to gain deeper contact with ourselves and to appreciate our own lives.

Mindfulness strengthens our capacity to be aware of the uniqueness and vitality of each moment. Through mindfulness we become more sensitive to our body sensations and to our deeply rooted, automatic patterns of thought and feeling. At the same time, being aware of our internal and external situation keeps us from becoming caught up in it. New space emerges in which we can observe problems from a distance and gain greater clarity for creative decision making and taking action.

At the beginning of the MBSR course, it is not possible to predict or promise exactly what will happen. However, experience has shown that being open to the richness of the present moment holds new and often unexpected possibilities for those prepared to discover them.

The following quote, which appeared in *Family Circle* magazine on March 27, 1978, is included in the course participant handbook and discussed at the end of Week 1. For many of our students it touches a soft place in their hearts and reminds them that everyday life is a treasure chest of mindful moments that only asks us to *look! look!*

If I had my life to live over, I'd dare to make more mistakes next time. I'd relax, I would limber up. I would be sillier than I have been this trip. I would take fewer things seriously. I would take more chances. I would climb more mountains and swim more rivers. I would eat more ice cream and less beans. I would perhaps have more actual troubles, but I'd have fewer imaginary ones.

You see, I'm one of those people who live sensibly and sanely, hour after hour, day after day. Oh, I've had my moments, and if I had to do it over again, I'd have more of them. In fact, I'd try to have nothing else. Just moments, one after another, instead of living so many years ahead of each day. I've been one of those persons who never goes anywhere without a thermometer, a hot water bottle, a raincoat and a parachute. If I had to do it again, I would travel lighter than I have.

If I had my life to live over, I would start barefoot earlier in the spring and stay that way later in the fall. I would go to more dances. I would ride more merry-go-rounds. I would pick more daisies.[20]

Tips for Mindful Eating

To begin with, it is generally easier to practice mindful eating in silence, rather than in conversation with other people. However, it is possible to practice in the company of others, and eventually you may wish to experiment with this. You might experiment with mindful eating for a whole meal or just a part of one. One mindfulness teacher suggests practicing mindful eating with the first bite of every meal. Sometimes when multiple people, including families, practice together, they eat mindfully in silence for the first five minutes of a meal.

- To begin with, look closely at whatever you are about to eat. What are its qualities in terms of color, shape, texture, smell, and so on?

- As you pick up the food, be aware of the fork or spoon in your hand and the sense of movement as you lift the food to your mouth.
- What do you notice as you place the food in your mouth? What does it feel like? What do you notice about its temperature, shape, size, and other qualities?
- Begin to chew slowly, being mindful of the taste of the food. Is it sweet, sour, tangy, bitter, spicy, bland, or something else? Take your time chewing and experiment with the amount of time that passes before you swallow.
- Be aware, as best you can, of the impulse to swallow. As you do swallow, notice any sensations that might be present as the food travels downward.
- Register each impulse to empty your mouth quickly to take the next bite.
- You might also try noticing how much you eat, how fast, how your body responds to the food, and what thoughts or emotions may be present.

WEEK 2

How We Perceive
the World and Ourselves

The real voyage of discovery consists not in seeking new landscapes but in having new eyes.

— Marcel Proust

In the second week of an MBSR class, we begin, after greeting one another, by lying down on the floor and being guided through a body scan. After the body scan, we take time to talk about what people experienced both in class and in practicing at home.

Here are some comments from participants about the body scan:

"I found myself constantly thinking about how I was going to find time to practice," said John. "It's quite funny as I talk about it now. All I needed to do was lie down and do it."

Barbara added a bit timidly, "The only thing I did during the body scan was fall asleep." (Several people smiled or nodded as she said this.)

Hans added, "I felt parts of my body I hadn't felt in years. It was good to connect to myself."

Joan, an older woman with severe arthritis, said, "Normally I do everything I can to distract myself from the pain. But I made the commitment to do the program, and I figured doing the body scan was part of it. During the scan, I kept coming back to wherever I was when my mind wandered. I noticed how much energy it takes in daily life when

I try to distract myself all the time. Maybe turning away is not always the answer."

Soon a particular question surfaces in the group: Is there a right way and a wrong way to do a body scan? In further discussion, people seem to agree that there is a tendency to think in the following way: "Right" means that people stay awake and feel relaxed afterward. "Wrong" means people fall asleep, or they feel more pain or discomfort.

The tendency to judge our experiences as right or wrong, good or bad, becomes immediately apparent when we practice mindfulness. This in itself is not bad or good, but sorting experiences into right ones and wrong ones has consequences: it causes many of us to shut ourselves off from a vast range of life events that do not fit into our scheme, and we subtly — and not so subtly — search for those things that will make us feel good and reject those that do not.

No Right, No Wrong

To help class participants explore their experience of the body scan, an MBSR teacher may ask questions like the following.

"What part of your body were you giving your attention to when you fell asleep?"

"What did you notice about the way you reacted when you realized you were drifting off and when you woke up?"

"You said at some point you thought this was boring. What was going on at the moment this thought came up?"

"I heard you say you did not experience a part of your body. Were you aware of any thoughts, feelings, or sensations at that time?"

"I understand that you're saying: at the end of the body scan, you felt a strong sense of your body as a whole, as if your breath were connecting the whole body. Can you say more about this?"

This art of inquiry about the body scan encourages us to investigate, sense, and be in contact with ourselves. This includes being aware of when we are not aware. It also communicates another very important understanding about the lessons of the body scan: *There is no right or wrong way to do a body scan.* Whatever experiences we have, they are valid exactly as they are. In such an exploration, we move from categorizing in absolute terms of right and wrong to savoring the rich nuance of every experience.

Is What You See What You Get?

The theme of Week 2 is becoming aware of how we perceive the world. In real terms, we explore the relationship between our interpretation of something and what is actually there. Most of us assume that the way we see things is the way they are, but nothing could be further from the truth. In a sense, we are always wearing glasses. Our lives — our backgrounds, cultures, personal histories, education, experiences, and all the people, ideas, and things that have influenced us — tint the lenses. Our attitudes, too, tint the lenses, and they filter what we perceive and influence the way we relate to the world.

What and how we see is very personal indeed. The opinions we form are just that: opinions. We often take them as absolute truth, and even though we can see a situation in a way completely unlike others do, down deep we think we are right and the others are mistaken.

Home Practice:
The Nine-Dot Exercise — How Attitudes Shape Perception

For home practice after Week 1, class members are asked to do the Nine-Dot Exercise.

The object of the exercise is to link up the nine dots using only four straight lines, without lifting the pen from the paper and without going twice over a line.

Comments about the Nine-Dot Exercise include the following:

- "I worked on it for three days, but I gave up after that. It's impossible to solve within the rules given."
- "I got frustrated quickly. And then I got angry. I felt sure something was missing from the explanation."
- "I found this to be a waste of time. I put it aside after the first five minutes."
- "I knew I had done this problem before. But I could not remember the solution. It drove me crazy."

The Nine-Dot Exercise seems to be unsolvable at first glance. The key to solving it lies in becoming aware that we often take assumptions to be true without questioning them, and that this leads to a limited view of a situation. Many participants experience an aha! moment when they finally see the answer to the puzzle. It then makes perfect sense that the answer can be found only by changing the way we see the problem.

In the lively discussions about the Nine-Dot Exercise that often take place, an understanding emerges about the tendency to get locked into one perspective. When we become aware of this, we've taken the first step toward shifting the way we perceive things.

Getting a Bigger Picture

In Week 2 of the MBSR course, the teacher may lead the mindful seeing exercise (see box on page 96).

On the lessons of mindful seeing, Dr. Nils Altner, who works as a mind-body therapist at the Clinic for Natural and Integrative Medicine at the University of Essen, Germany, writes,

A key aspect of being mindful in facing stress is to be aware of a situation that we may not be able to change, but where we may very well be able to change the nature of our perception. When we are stressed, we often see things from only one perspective. The practice of mindful seeing can help us see how to expand our own ideas about the world or contract them. By seeing the whole picture and being aware of more of the finer details of that picture, it is as if we were trying on a new pair of glasses for the first time.

We could continue to cope with the old glasses, but the new ones allow us to see so much sharper and clearer and with more detail. We could, of course, live with the old glasses and simply miss the opportunity to see better with the new ones. However, with respect to our own situation, we have a choice. With mindful seeing it's all about making this choice as if it were a gift of seeing clearly, a gift that we can give to ourselves, motivated by a caring and friendly attitude.

When we focus our perception on something, we naturally have opinions about it, such as "That's wonderful" or "That's not for me" or "I've seen everything" or "This is nothing new" and so on. If I look around without an actual target for my gaze, unexpected things can happen. A very focused view will reveal something different to an open, unfocused view — a telephoto lens as opposed to a wide-angle lens.

The nine-point exercise and the mindful seeing exercise [see next page] show us that we can shape how we perceive a situation and, in so doing, see new perspectives or even solutions that we have not seen before.[21]

Mindful Seeing Exercise

The mindful seeing exercise explores how we direct our gaze and selective sight. It is best to practice mindful seeing in a room with a large window, ideally one that allows a view of the outdoors. Or you can practice outside. A quiet atmosphere is supportive. The exercise can take anywhere from ten to twenty minutes. The following version is based on instructions given by Dr. Altner in his MBSR classes.[22]

- Begin by looking out the window. Let your gaze wander, noticing the entire picture framed by the window: the individual objects, houses, trees, people, and so on. Experiment with perceiving the foreground...middle ground...background...the surfaces and colors.
- Helpful questions to ask yourself include:
  - Which thoughts arise when I look in this way?
  - What emotions or moods am I aware of, if any?

- Now, focus your gaze on a small area. How do you perceive what surrounds this area (or point)? What happens to the rest of the picture when you focus as exclusively as you can on this area?
- After spending time gazing like this, let your focus soften by allowing your eye muscles to relax and your gaze to blur. After a time, begin experimenting with shifting your gaze in various ways. For example:
  - Can you expand the area of your gaze until it encompasses the entire vista?
  - Can you change the focus of your attention without moving your eyes, or are your focus and your eyes linked?
  - What are you aware of (thoughts, sensations, emotions) now that your attention is spread evenly over the entire vista?

- • What do you notice if you now focus laserlike on a new point?
- Continue to play with the focus of your gaze by experimenting with the following:
  - • Without moving your head, can you see parts of yourself? For example: your nose ... your glasses ... your upper lip?
  - • Experiment with turning your attention inward, but continue to keep your eyes open. Do you sense your breath? Your body? Are you aware of thoughts or feelings or both?
- Continue to experiment with gazing around the room but staying focused internally. Look at the various objects in the room.
- Now become aware of your own body as strongly as you can as you continue to look at the scene in front of you.
  - • Do you sense your breath? Your body?
  - • Are you aware of thoughts? Feelings?
  - • What happens to your gaze when you direct your attention inward?
  - • Can you feel the physical sensations of breathing?
  - • How does your breath move your body?
- Continue to keep your awareness completely on yourself ... on your breathing and on your body. At the same time, allow your gaze to wander among the various objects in the room.
- After some time, let go of focusing your gaze on objects and slowly end the exercise. Next, you may want to close your eyes to rest them. Then move, stretch, yawn, or do anything else your body seems to ask for.

The mindful seeing exercise helps underline the possibility that we can change the way we perceive events in our lives and, in doing so, reshape our whole experience of an event. Irmgard's story, for example, illustrates how her perception of a difficult experience in the past transformed into a source of wisdom for dealing with present-day challenges:

> When I was around six years old, I walked into a basement to get my bicycle. The light was broken, but there was some sunlight visible through the dirty window. At some point I thought I saw a shadow of a man, who seemed to be holding a gun. I ran out of the cellar. To this day I don't know whether there was someone there or not.
>
> I came to MBSR because I have a lot of fears...about my work, my children, and just life in general. The practice of mindfulness helped me to get in touch with some of my fears. I learned to be with the uncomfortable sensations, thoughts, or feelings that came up. Now when I worry about something, especially when I am challenged, I tell myself, "It's time to go and get the bike out of the basement."
>
> I may not be able to get rid of the initial fear that comes up, but I can be aware of it so that it no longer limits where I go and what I do. My fear is still there, but it no longer stops me. Sometimes, it is even like a friend, supporting me when I am about to give up. A very dear friend, indeed.

Home Practice: Lessons of Mindful Breathing

As part of the home practice following Week 2, participants are asked to practice an awareness-of-breath meditation. This meditation is one that many participants continue to practice years after the course is over.

Have you ever noticed how the breath changes according to your moods: short and shallow when you are tense or angry, faster when you are excited, steady and strong when you are happy, and almost absent when you are scared? Our breath is with us all the time. If we make a practice of being aware of our breath, we can use it to anchor and stabilize the body and mind in the present. We can tune in to our breath at any given moment.

We are not in touch with our breathing most of the time. This is why one of the first mindfulness exercises in MBSR is to connect with the breath. We don't need to control our breath; we just want to be aware of it as best we can and get to know it as we would a friend.

Mindful breathing teaches us that it is possible to be present in each inhalation and exhalation, breath by breath. It helps us to anchor ourselves in the here and now, to experience the present moment to the fullest. At the same time, it demonstrates that mindfulness is not a permanent state but one established again and again. Returning the attention to the breath each time we notice we have drifted away is a powerful step toward sustaining wakefulness as well as the practice of meticulous attention in our lives.

Many people find that the subtle confidence derived from being able to come back to the present moment through mindful breathing is nurturing and self-affirming. It affirms that we can be in touch with and flow with the moments of our lives rather than drift aimlessly.

We also can see in mindful breathing (as we did in the body scan) how judgmental we can be about ourselves and how strong our need is to be right. When we notice that the mind is no longer focused on the breath, it is easy to get caught up in various mental responses. We may judge or criticize ourselves, make comments such as "It's too hard," or start laughing at the absurdity of it all.

Cultivating friendliness toward ourselves and a gentle recognition of the harshness that springs up within us is a step toward healing. Rather than focusing on getting it right or meeting a standard, we affirm, breath by breath, that life can flow, especially when we get out of the way and allow it to just be.

Our inner attitude toward ourselves is just as important in meditation as knowing how to follow the instructions. Our attitude affects our practice. If we have the impression that meditation is a test to pass, we make it an unpleasant duty. If we are too focused on relaxing, we may become tense or very tired and then disappointed when we cannot relax.

Exercise: Mindful Breathing

These instructions are designed to guide you through the practice of mindful breathing. There are several ways to work with them:

1. You can read the text, pausing at the end of each section.
2. You can read the whole text first, possibly several times, and then practice mindful breathing for a certain time without looking at the text.

If sitting meditation is new to you, we suggest that at first you practice for ten minutes at a time.

*   Chose whichever sitting aid is comfortable for you — a chair, kneeling bench, or meditation cushion, or sit up in bed.
*   Sit as best you can in an upright, relaxed position. Gently drop your chin downward toward your chest, so that you feel a very slight stretching and elongation at the back of your neck. Rest your hands on your thighs, or fold them into each other in your lap — whatever is most comfortable. You may either close your eyes or leave them open and gaze softly downward.
*   Take a moment to experience the body while sitting. Tune in to your body, experiencing any sensations you may be aware of. These could include the contact between your sitz bones and the surface you are seated on or the contact of your hands, either with each other or with your thighs.
*   Bring your attention to the sensations of breathing. It is helpful to direct your awareness to the part of the body where you feel the breath most clearly. Perhaps it is in the abdomen; if so, sense its expansion and release as you inhale...and exhale. Perhaps you feel your breath

more in the upper part of your body — the ribs and lungs moving with every cycle of breathing. Perhaps you feel your breath most clearly at the edges of your nostrils as you notice the air stream in and out. Maybe there is another area of the body where you feel the sensations of breathing most vividly.

- Pick one of these areas of the body and stay with it for the rest of the exercise.
- Be aware of the sensations as your breath flows into the body...and as it flows out. Just allow your breath to come and go, as it does of its own accord.
- You may notice from time to time that you want the breath to be different from the way it is. Just notice that this thought has come up, then gently and clearly direct your attention back to the flow of breath in and out of the body.
- You might also notice that you comment on the process — either positively or negatively. For example: "I'm doing this particularly well today" or "This exercise just doesn't work for me." As soon as you become aware of these comments just note to yourself: "This is just a thought." Then turn your attention back to your breath with a friendly and curious attitude. No judging, no self-criticism is necessary. Just gently come back to the breath.
- Feel how one breath follows the other. Perhaps you can also be aware of the pause between breaths.
- As you practice, you may notice your attention wandering, whether you're caught up in a daydream or a memory. You may be making plans for the future or worrying about something. If you notice this, then pause for a moment and note where your thoughts have

drifted to — for example: "I'm planning my next shopping trip" or "I'm worrying about a conversation with my colleague."

- It is entirely natural that our attention drifts. In mindfulness practice, we do not consider this a problem or a failure on our part. We observe the tendency to wander, as we notice everything else, and then return to the sensations of breathing.

- Be with your breathing, breath for breath, as it is at this moment, without controlling or judging it.

- If you are aware of tension in the body, see if it is possible to let your awareness soften. It may be helpful to lighten the focus on your breathing.

- If your awareness is too soft, however, you may find that you are drifting off or feeling sleepy. If you notice this, then bring your attention back to the sensation of breathing.

- At the same time, awaken your curiosity about the breath. Are the breaths long or short? Are they on the surface or deeper in the body? Drifting can also be a result of going on automatic pilot, and so we support ourselves by bringing our interest and a sense of vitality to the breathing process.

- Observe the sensations that are present when breathing in...and breathing out.

- From time to time, direct your attention to your posture and how you are seated. Perhaps you are pitched forward or your shoulders are raised. Maybe your upper body is slightly slumped or leaning to one side. If this is the case, then you may mindfully alter your position. If you move, do it as a mindfulness exercise by being aware of all the sensations of movement and the changes in your body. If we move in this way, which is similar to the way we experience the postures in yoga, then it becomes mindful movement.

- Just be with the breath...and the next breath...and the next...
- When you decide to end the exercise, take a few moments to sit quietly. After that, stretch a little and perhaps gently massage your temples or move your shoulders, hands, or feet. Stand up gradually and walk slowly in a relaxed way for a short time.

WEEK 3

Being at Home
in Our Own Body

A journey of discovery that began with the body scan continues, in Week 3, with yoga. One focus of the third session of the MBSR course is learning a series of gentle yoga exercises to practice at home. Katharina Meinhard, a teacher in our institute, described yoga's role in MBSR like this:

> Many people have a distorted image of their body and its possibilities. With simple movements and postures, mindful yoga can help us to become aware of these misperceptions and we notice how old patterns of movement and thought sabotage our physical, emotional, and mental health.
>
> Yoga promotes body awareness, strength, flexibility, and coordination. Body and breath can be experienced anew in a fresh way. Fostering a kind attitude toward ourselves, and the gaze of beginner's mind, in yoga we cultivate self-acceptance, patience, and trust.
>
> There is no distant goal we wish to attain — as we are now, we are unique, complete, and whole. To acknowledge and appreciate this will open us up to the wonder of the present moment, and we take a step further toward integration and wholeness.[23]

Coming Home to Yourself

What many people discover during yoga practice (and earlier in the body scan) is that we are rarely at home in our bodies. Most of the time we are up in our heads. Whether at work, in everyday life, or even in the quiet moments when we are apparently relaxing, our minds are busy with thoughts, plans, memories, or problems to solve. We often stay in our heads until something happens. It could be when we receive a diagnosis of illness, or are in an accident, or become aware of pain. Suddenly sensations of the body arise, along with strong emotions like anger, rejection, or shame.

Karin, a thirty-eight-year-old woman diagnosed with multiple sclerosis, told the group in the first meeting of the course: "When I found out I had MS, I was so angry at my body. I could no longer do things the way I used to. I love to surf, but I didn't have the strength to get up on the board. I could no longer trust my body. I was so disappointed and frustrated." Karin's comments moved many of the people in her class, not only because she shared her feelings but also because they recognized themselves in her words. A first reaction that many people have when they become ill is to feel as if their bodies have betrayed them. They may experience anger, fear, frustration, regret, and a whole host of disturbing emotions and thoughts. Often it is not a time when we can readily hear comforting words; the sense of loss is too strong.

Karin continued with her story:

I signed up for an MBSR class because I wanted to come to terms with myself. I knew I would never be able to surf again. Even harder to face were all my negative and judgmental thoughts about myself.

But now sometimes, underneath all the harshness, I hear a more gentle voice that says, "Come on, Karin! You love to be in the ocean. Let that be the joy that you give to yourself."

In every moment, whatever the condition of our health, we are living, breathing, and continuing to show up for life. There is something powerful about this fact; it has the same energy that allows a seed to germinate in spring after a winter in hibernation.

When we become ill or the demands of overextending ourselves take their toll, our lives may no longer include all our previous activities. Nevertheless, life still calls out to us in every moment: "Are you here? Are you present?" There is another question, one whispered softly: *"Are you willing to entertain the possibility that your present situation is not the end but the beginning of a new phase of your life?"* If so, mindfulness practice can support you as you let go of the life that was, so that you can live the life that is.

Yoga: Mindfulness of Boundaries

In practicing yoga, the theme of encountering boundaries often arises as we explore our physical experience of the exercises and our reactions to them. In general, many people are not aware of their boundaries, either because they constantly go beyond them or because they hesitate to approach them. Sometimes we find a movement difficult and back off from doing it; other times we push ourselves to stretch further and further, beyond what might be suitable for us at this time. Sometimes we are so preoccupied with the effort that we lose contact with our bodies completely.

The word *boundary* often has a negative connotation. It implies that something is limited or forbidden. The usual advice for working with boundaries is to "break through" or "push beyond." Yet not honoring our boundaries can result in forcing ourselves past what is good for us.

Becoming aware of our boundaries, on the other hand, is an invitation to sit up and take notice. Boundaries invite us to care for ourselves. They open us to new levels of sensitivity that ask us to come in close, to explore carefully and tenderly. Being in tune with our bodies can help us be in tune with ourselves, and this encourages us to ask, "What nurtures me?"

In mindfulness practice, we discover that boundaries can shift and change. Rather than break through them, we can explore them.

Later in the course, Karin told us more about her shifting attitude toward herself:

Last week I tried to climb up on my surfboard again. My husband watched me struggle, and I could see my pain mirrored in his eyes. After trying at least six times, I was exhausted. I gave up and floated on my back for a very long time. All the tension drained away, as if the ocean were absorbing it. I felt such peace.

Suddenly, I realized that I could still surf. Not on top of my board, but alongside it. I felt the ocean now in a way I never had before.... This may sound a bit corny, but before, I used to surf the waves. Now I am the wave itself.

Yoga as Tuning In to Ourselves

In yoga, we practice tuning in to sensations in the same way we did in the body scan. As we begin to explore sensations and their different layers of intensity, we can notice that they consist of different qualities.

Sensations can include qualities of lightness, heaviness, warmth, cold, tickling, or prickling, to name only a few. The sensations that we notice can vary from day to day, even from hour to hour or breath to breath. We may experience a relaxation of muscular tension, lightness, or a stronger sense of grounding. We may also experience tightness, burning, or pulsation — some sensations may be pleasant, some may be unpleasant. And this, too, can change from moment to moment.

If you are coming to yoga with a history of chronic pain, you may become aware of your pain in a way that you never have before. This does not necessarily mean you have more pain, only that you are more aware of it. At first there can be a sense of disappointment or confusion, especially if you are determined to get rid of discomfort. But as your mindfulness practice continues, you may become aware that you let go of results and just quietly ask from moment to moment: "And what is this? And this? And this?"

Helpful Hints for Practicing Yoga in MBSR

Practicing yoga is not about achieving something or only being concerned about how to perform the exercises. Practicing yoga mindfully is about becoming aware of ourselves and what we are experiencing in the moment. Questions that can help us be mindful include: "What is happening right now?" "What am I sensing?" and "What do I notice?"

We practice being aware of the sensations we feel as we notice whether they are getting stronger or weaker. We also observe our reactions to the sensations. For example, when you observe yourself, do you feel stable and calm? Do you notice restlessness and have thoughts darting here and there? Try to become aware of everything that happens, but without changing, adding, or omitting anything. You may notice, however, that you try to do so anyway. As best you can, pay attention to this as you practice, to just being with what is, from moment to moment.

When practicing yoga, it's important to respect what is possible on any given day. If you sense that doing an exercise is not good for you or perhaps not possible that day, then not doing it is a way of taking care of yourself; pushing through is exactly the opposite. If you decide not to do an exercise, then take a comfortable position, close your eyes, and do the exercise as thoroughly as you can in your mind's eye. You also have the option of modifying an exercise and working with your abilities. The teacher will be glad to explore alternatives with you.

We've discussed the idea that yoga is about exploring boundaries, but how exactly do we accomplish this? For example, when you stretch within a posture, you may notice that you're thinking you should end the stretch. You may notice that you stop before any sense of discomfort appears. You may then notice that you are stopping before it is necessary. On the other hand, you may notice that you sense a need to go further, and that in an effort to do so, you push yourself beyond what is helpful or healthy for your body. Raise the intention to take care of yourself, and see if it is possible to refrain from following the impulse that is arising. Then, return to the yoga posture and continue.

We can learn a great deal about our body, mind, and heart through yoga practice. We can apply those lessons to living mindfully: discovering the space between doing too much and doing too little, we find the way of doing just enough. We learn to trust the wisdom of asking, "What is the best way for me?"

Becoming Aware of Our Relationships to Sensation, Including Pain

One frequent reaction to pain is resistance, which often takes the form of the body tightening up in anticipation or reaction. Mentally, too, we may tighten up, or we may try to distract ourselves.

When asked to describe a sensation, we tend to do so in terms of our emotional reaction to it. We like it…or we don't like it…or are indifferent. There can be multiple reactions to the same situation. For athletes, having sore muscles after exertion is something they are accustomed to. They also know that stretching properly will increase flexibility and improve performance. For people with a chronic pain condition, experiencing tight muscles or soreness may be a sign that the condition is worsening — and they may fear stretching because the pain may get worse.

How can it be helpful to know the distinction between describing a sensation as objectively as possible and having an emotional reaction to it? When I (Petra) present this question in MBSR classes, some participants look at me skeptically. Some say strongly, "Pain is pain!" Others say, "It sounds like you are saying I have to accept the pain. But isn't it natural to want to get rid of it?"

As the course proceeds, participants confirm for themselves what many tell us they discover: there is no guarantee that discomfort will end, but we can change our relationship to it. The shift includes moving from being a victim to being an active witness.

Shinzen Young, an American meditation teacher who has worked with many chronic pain patients, describes the relationship between pain and resistance as follows:

> For example, an uncomfortable sensation may arise in your knee as you're meditating. At the same time, you may observe that in reaction to the pain, you are clenching and tightening other parts of your body, while in your mind a stream of judgments and aversive thoughts [is] erupting.
>
> The sensation in your knee is the pain. The tension is your bodily resistance. The judgments are mental resistance. The resistance can be distinguished clearly from the pain itself. As you consciously relax the tension and drop the judgments, even though the pain level is the same, it seems to be less of a problem.... You are making your first steps in learning how to experience pain skillfully.[24]

As It Is, It's Okay

For someone who is used to pushing to excel, the statement "As it is, it's okay" does not compute. For them, it's simply not an option that can be entertained even briefly. It sounds too much like passive acceptance of things as they are. Their modus operandi is to see each situation as a challenge to overcome, with clenched jaw and all.

Yoga is a field of practice where we can recognize this form of supposed self-encouragement as disguised self-judgment. We can learn that our self-worth is independent of how successful we are with the yoga exercises. Acknowledging the truth of the moment in yoga, as in life, broadens our mind and opens our heart. If we are stiff one morning and we rest rather than push beyond a certain point, a soft thank-you can arise within us, not so much in words but in a gentle ease that settles in our body.

In both yoga and the body scan, we become aware of our body as a complex sensing organ that is continually evolving. As we become aware of the impermanence of all things, including our body, we can experience a sense of tenderness toward the fragile organism that is us. Through mindfulness we can come to recognize that change is not an obstacle but an indicator of potential. This helps us live a full life *with* pain rather than in spite of it.

Many participants in an MBSR course find it possible to live with difficulties and pain without trying to get rid of them or change things. The battles they fight within themselves abate as a sense of self-acceptance grows. Others who once felt that they were unable to do yoga see that they are capable of more than they imagined. The glass is no longer half empty but half full and, sometimes, even on the verge of overflowing.

Mindfulness practice can help release us from the prison of perfection into the tender beauty of our imperfect — and wonderful — bodies and lives.

What Is Stress?

The fourth week of the MBSR program usually begins with a guided sitting meditation. We consider in greater depth how mindfulness training can help us handle difficult situations and cope more effectively with what we experience as stress in our lives — which is also a theme for this session.

Through practice, we find that our ability to be mindful of our breathing strengthens. This is by no means as easy as it sounds. In our daily meditation practice we soon notice how hard it is to really rest our attention on the breath. When practicing, we may worry about pain in our legs, or thoughts may flood the mind in the form of memories, plans, hopes, or fears. Often, one of them will capture our attention to such an extent that it's a long time before we notice we've lost touch with the breath. Full of determination and optimism, we start over, only to realize after a few moments that our thoughts have drifted off again. We may well ask, "Who is actually in charge here?"

From the moment we begin to practice mindfulness, it becomes apparent that we drift easily into being unfocused and unaware. Like a child demanding a toy and then tiring of it, then wanting another and yet another, our mind jumps from one thought — one object of awareness — to another. With regular mindfulness practice, we begin to see that we can train and calm our restless mind.

It is helpful for class participants to share their meditation experiences with each other as well as receive support and guidance from the teacher. Otherwise, it's all too easy to become discouraged by ideas such as: "Meditation just won't work for me" or "I'll never be able to do this; I just keep getting distracted and becoming more and more restless."

We need patience at this point to accept that observing and acknowledging our restless mind is part of the mindfulness journey. Wandering off track, and observing that we have done so, is as much a part of mindfulness meditation as calmly dwelling on the object of our awareness. We can notice over time that the more we practice mindfulness, the more our thoughts tend to slow down. In particular, we may find that random trains of thought no longer derail us quite so often. We tend to recognize earlier: "Ah, here comes a thought, but I don't have to follow it. My intent now is to stay focused on my breathing."

One course participant expressed it this way: "If I notice that my mind is restless and my thoughts are jumping back and forth, I say to them in a friendly way: 'You can go wherever you like, but I am staying right here.'"

Body and Breath

Practicing mindful breathing will help us become more aware of our body and how we relate to the world around us. Thus, once we have developed some ability to be mindful of the breath, we turn our awareness to mindfulness of the body. At first, we become aware of our body as a whole, and then we tune in to our awareness of bodily sensations. We perceive the sensations as impartially as we can and just observe them as they make themselves felt. At the same time, by being aware of physical sensations, we learn not to react right away, regardless of whether the sensations are pleasant, unpleasant, or neutral. Later in this book, we will show how this can be helpful for stress reduction.

Mindfulness Exercise: Awareness of Breathing, the Body, and Its Sensations

- As always, start the exercise with awareness of the sitting posture, taking time to find an upright and comfortable position. Then center the awareness on a part of the body where you most clearly feel the breath — it might be the tip of the nose, the rib cage, the abdominal region, or any other part of the body. Practice mindful breathing as taught earlier.

- Wandering off into thought may happen often. Each time you recognize that it has happened, as patiently and gently as possible return your awareness to the breath.

- Sometimes a particular expectation — or the desire for something specific, such as a pleasant experience or the ability to get rid of an unpleasant one — will be present. If this happens, see if it is possible to observe the expectation itself without being caught up in it. You may notice that this expectation generates tension in your mind and body. See if it is possible to let go of the expectation itself and continue to sit and observe what is arising without intervening in any way.

- Next, when you are ready, expand your attention to include the body as a whole. Perhaps you sense the form of your whole body and the space it takes up. Maybe you sense your body's boundary: the skin. You may become aware of physical sensations such as pressure, tingling, strain, or itching. Allow, as best you can, your awareness to remain lightly focused on these sensations for as long as they make themselves felt. Then, when they lessen in intensity, return your awareness back to the body as a whole — sitting as you are at this very moment.

- There's no need to force yourself to feel sensations in a certain way or to go looking for them. Remain aware of the body as best you can and observe from moment to moment what arises.

- As the meditation draws to a close, bring your attention back to the breath, being aware of it as it comes and goes, one breath after the other. Then, whenever you are ready, end the meditation in your own way.

The mood during the fourth session can be ambivalent. Course participants notice that as they go about daily activities, their capacity to focus on one thing at a time has improved as mindfulness establishes itself. At the same time, however, some notice that they are more aware than before of unpleasant sensations, pain, problems, and stress signals.

As we have mentioned already, through practicing mindfulness we become more aware of things that we were unconscious of, or less conscious of, previously. These include pleasant, joyful, and gratifying events, as well as adverse personal circumstances, difficult situations, and painful sensations.

Developing more awareness is one of the keys to how mindfulness helps us cope with stress in a skillful way. For in order to make changes that lead to reducing stress, we first need to know what is going on. When we do, we can better explore what needs to be changed and what might be necessary to accomplish it.

If we are sick and go to a doctor, he or she will start by examining us and then will make a diagnosis. Based on the diagnosis, the doctor will recommend suitable treatment. What the doctor definitely will *not* do is advise us to ignore our illness. Similarly, it is important for us to explore the source of our stress and exactly how it affects our lives and our health. Initially, this is bound to be unfamiliar and uncomfortable, because we tend to avoid disagreeable experiences and sensations rather than meet them head-on.

It may help to recall the discussion of stress in chapter 3. When we are under stress, the fight-or-flight response is automatically triggered, which means we try to avoid, get rid of, or nullify the cause of stress and any emotions produced by it. We sense that we are agitated, anxious, and in turmoil, but we find it hard to stay with whatever is coming up without intervening. In the past, we may have tried to reduce the intensity of these emotions by, for example, blaming others or indulging in certain behaviors such as self-medication. We are unaccustomed, however, to mindfully staying present for what emerges from inside. Though this would be much more helpful in the long run than fighting or trying to suppress parts of ourselves, we are not at home with this approach.

Our internal pressure to solve problems and get rid of unpleasantness is very powerful. In this fourth session of the course, we look at this in more detail. As we do so, it becomes clearer why it is helpful to acknowledge our problems and stay with whatever emotions or thoughts are arising, rather than blindly reacting to them or denying them. For when we deny our (unpleasant) experiences, the pattern of avoidance creates a — mostly unconscious — fear. This fear becomes a stress trigger in itself. So denying unpleasant experiences ultimately produces internalized chronic stress for the body. Mindfulness is about learning how we can turn toward the unpleasant and be with it.

For many participants the fourth session is a turning point. They begin to understand more deeply what mindfulness is and why interrupting the automatic pilot mode of behavior is helpful. It also becomes more apparent why MBSR is not a quick fix to get rid of stress but rather a path to reduce the experience of stress by changing the way we relate to our life in the first place.

Stress is a part of our lives, just as there is night and day. We can't change that. What we can change is how we relate to our experiences and how we cope with stress. That is what we will focus on in the remaining sessions. Each course participant will be seeking his or her own answer to a fundamental question: How can I learn to relate to the situations in my life that I experience as stressful so that I can cope with them skillfully and not let them get the better of me?

At this stage in the course, the teacher will give a brief talk on stress, the various theories surrounding it, and how it affects our health (see chapter 3). In this context, it's important to identify our own personal stress triggers and to recognize the signs of stress in ourselves. We start by learning to recognize the early warning signs that show us we need to take action in order to avoid getting caught up in a stress cycle. The body scan and mindful yoga are valuable tools in this respect because they help us become aware of sensations. Physical sensations in turn can be warning signs of stress: they can include feeling more tired than usual, muscular tension, digestive problems, headaches, neck or back pain, among others. These physical stress signals will vary from person to person. What matters, however, is that mindfulness training can help us recognize stress triggers and stress reactions and become more aware of the early warning signals of both.

Through mindfulness training and an enhanced awareness of our bodies, thoughts, and emotions, we can become familiar with which situations trigger stress. In this way, we also become more aware of our habitual coping and assessment strategies. What helps us develop more awareness is a "mindful pause." If we pause, we can develop the capacity to turn toward rather than turn away. Eventually, this sensitivity to all aspects of the stress situation and our individual stress reactions can lead to a new way of dealing with them. The result is no longer an automatic reaction or avoidance mechanism. Other creative solutions can arise from mindfully pausing and being aware of where we are (emotionally, cognitively, physically) at that moment. Ultimately, this enables us to think, feel, and act in a way that is physically and emotionally healthier.

In Week 4, we continue to develop our ability to observe and be aware without judgment. In Week 5, we will look at how to be mindful in relation to unconscious judgments and stress-provoking thoughts. To prepare at home for Week 5, carefully observe personal stress triggers and stress reactions without making any changes. It's not an easy task, but certainly a worthwhile one.

WEEK 5

Stress: Reaction or Mindful Response

It is not what we experience but how we perceive it that defines our destiny.

— Marie von Ebner-Eschenbach

In Week 5 we usually start the class with a longer sitting meditation. We begin as usual by adopting an upright and relaxed posture and then turn our attention to our breath. From there, in the course of the meditation, our awareness expands to encompass our bodies as a whole and any physical sensations that may arise moment by moment. In the next step, we direct our attention to the sense of hearing (see box on page 122).

When practicing mindful listening on its own, you can end the meditation by bringing the awareness back to the breath and resting in stillness for some time before starting your daily activity. In Week 5 of the course, however, we do not stop with mindful hearing but continue by becoming aware of our thought process and then the emotions. Just as sounds come and go, so do thoughts and emotions: they appear, stay for a while, and then move on.

In the sitting meditation, we practice purposely observing thoughts and emotions without changing, judging, or personally identifying with them. The thoughts could be about anything. They can be about the past, present, or future. They can include plans, memories, ideas, or wishes. They can be pleasant, unpleasant, or neutral. Whatever or however they are, we just observe them, as best we can, as simply mental activity. As we continue the meditation, mindfulness of thoughts and emotions recedes to the background and we rest for some time in what is called "choiceless awareness" (see box on facing page).

Mindfulness Exercise: Mindful Hearing

- Sit in a comfortable upright position. When you feel settled in the posture, become aware of your sense of hearing. Allow any sounds that may be present to come to your ears of their own accord.

- Don't strain to hear any sounds in particular. Register these sounds as best you can without trying to name or rate them. They may be noises from inside your body, inside the room, or from outside.

- If you find yourself identifying or assessing the sounds, or if certain associations come to mind when you hear them, this is perfectly normal. Be aware of these reactions for what they are: thoughts, memories, associations, or images. Then, return to just listening. Explore whether it is possible to listen without deciding whether you like the sounds or not. You may also try exploring the space between the sounds.

- Allow yourself to experience your sense of hearing as best you can, from one moment to the next. Spend a few minutes practicing in this way.

- If you wish, you may end the mindful hearing exercise here. You may return either to awareness of breathing or to a sense of the body sitting. You might also continue to the next meditation on choiceless awareness.

Mindfulness Exercise:
The Practice of Choiceless Awareness

In the practice of choiceless awareness, we observe what arises without focusing our attention on anything in particular. We practice being aware of various phenomena such as sounds, thoughts, emotions, sensations, and the breath as they arise from moment to moment:

- ◆ When you sense the breath, then experience the breath.
- ◆ When you feel sensations, be mindful of them.
- ◆ When you hear sounds, just listen.
- ◆ When thoughts or emotions arise, just notice that they are there.

Let's begin:

- Continue to sit and witness the rising and fading away of each of these phenomena without attaching yourself to it or distancing yourself from it. By doing so, you are bearing witness to the flow of life from moment to moment that includes all these objects of awareness.
- It may be that from time to time you find yourself caught up in a thought, emotion, sound, or sensation. You may find yourself thinking about it or trying in some way to influence it. When you notice this, just acknowledge that your awareness has fixed on an object, and then widen your awareness to take in the present moment in its fullness, where all objects come and go without one being more prominent than another.
- To end the meditation, return to practicing awareness of breathing. If you wish, you may remind yourself of the possibility to practice choiceless awareness in everyday life: being in the moment as it unfolds, present for what is.

Choiceless Awareness

What exactly is choiceless awareness? How can practicing it help us cope with stress?

Through choiceless awareness, we acknowledge everything that is present without having any particular expectations or preferences. We just observe the ebb and flow of our emotions, thoughts, physical sensations, or mental images as they come and go. Our awareness takes on the quality of a mirror that reflects whatever we hold up to it without attempting to alter it. In this manner, we cultivate a mind-set that helps us to both remain composed even in times of stress and face whatever happens. We can even perceive fear — the feeling of "How am I ever going to get through this?" — as just another facet (a thought, in fact) of the life experience. In this way, we begin to strengthen mindful presence in the face of challenging situations.

Viewing Thoughts in a New Way

It's not what happens to you, but how you react to it, that matters.

— Epictetus

On conclusion of the sitting meditation at the beginning of the fifth week, the participants share their experiences of it. They address in particular the question of how we can observe our thought processes without becoming involved in their contents. Interestingly, many participants report that when they observe their thoughts during meditation, these thoughts seem to vanish. Take, for example, the experience of Britta.

Britta told the class: "I found it amazing. Normally I spend the whole day just thinking, thinking, thinking. I feel totally weighed down by this constant mental chatter. I just can't switch it off, even though I know it's not doing me any good. Just now, though, when I tried to analyze my worries during the meditation, they were suddenly gone. How is that possible?"

Asked how she noticed that the thoughts had disappeared, Britta answered, "There just weren't any, though there's usually so many."

The teacher then asked her how she knew there were no thoughts. Britta replied, "I don't know, I just noticed it."

The teacher continued: "Britta, can it be that at first there was a sort of break in your thinking, and then you thought something along the lines of: 'Hey, the worries have stopped?'"

"Yes, that's exactly how it was!"

The teacher then asked, "Was it clear to you in that moment that the idea '*Hey! There are no thoughts*' was itself a thought?"

Britta appeared confused for a moment, and then said, "No, that wasn't clear to me. But looking back, it's obvious. That's a tricky one — I really didn't notice it at the time."

What did Britta mean by *tricky*? Her experience shows in fact how subtle the power of our thoughts is, and how entangled we are in them. If our minds really do go blank for a few seconds, then invariably we find ourselves conscious of an absence of thoughts — and there we are again, back in thinking mode.

Meditation is not about clearing our minds of thoughts — a common misconception — but about recognizing a thought for what it is and then letting it go. This can eventually lead to the realization *I am not my thoughts; I have thoughts.*

Many people who take an MBSR course describe this as one of the most important and valuable insights of the whole program. The power of this understanding lies in the fact that it opens up the possibility of choice: we can decide which thoughts we want to believe and which we do not. We can notice the effect that different kinds of thoughts have on us, and how mindfulness can shift our relationship to them.

Klaus had an important understanding in relation to this. He took part in an MBSR course because he suffered from recurring mood swings and wanted to learn how to deal with his negative thoughts in particular, which he found hard to shrug off. He reported that this insight into the nature of thinking and thoughts was the single most important discovery he had made during the course.

In the past, I woke up with negative thoughts like: "Oh, I just don't feel like getting up. It's all hopeless anyway. There's no way I'll manage to do everything I intend to do today, so I may as well not even bother trying. And what if I feel just as bad tomorrow; where will it all end?"

I then felt so bad that I just stayed in bed. But that didn't make me feel any better either; it made me feel like a failure — depressed and ill.

Now I know that when I have these thoughts, they're nothing but thoughts. I register them mindfully, and they don't feel good, but I don't allow them to get the upper hand anymore....I observe the thoughts, just the way we practice doing it in our meditation sessions here, and then I get up and start my day. I usually end up feeling better. For me that's groundbreaking. I am free to decide whether to get up or not. It has totally revolutionized my quality of life.

In the previous chapter, we invited you to examine your own stress triggers and experiences. Perhaps you noted how stress affected your body and well-being, as well as your reactions when exposed to stress. By pausing mindfully, by breathing and being in the moment, it is possible to create a space between a stress trigger and the ensuing reaction, which usually occurs immediately and automatically. We find that this awareness of a space between the trigger and the stress reaction can influence not only our experience of a situation but its outcome as well.

Exploring Stress-Increasing Thoughts

At this point in the course, our focus shifts to seeing how mindfulness can help us deal with stress in a way that mitigates its negative impact on our health. As described above, the first step is to pause for a moment to identify both the stress trigger and our reaction to it, and to recognize the early warning signs of stress. The formal MBSR exercises, including the body scan, yoga, and sitting meditation, all strengthen this capacity to stay in touch with our bodies and recognize the early signs of stress.

The next stage is about discovering what happens on the cognitive level — at the level of our thoughts, judgments, and emotions — when we feel stressed. We can't banish stress from our lives entirely, but we can influence how we deal with it by evaluating the stress-amplifying thoughts that play a major role.

Largely, stress and burdensome emotions begin in our minds. Research indicates that we can make a significant contribution toward coping with stress by identifying our stress triggers and stress-amplifying thoughts (see, for example, Richard S. Lazarus and Susan Folkman's *Stress, Appraisal, and Coping*).[25] As a rule, our assessments and value judgments occur instantly. If we can be aware of these in a calm and friendly manner — as practiced in mindfulness meditation — and then allow them to move on instead of giving them credence or identifying with them, they gradually lose their harmful impact on us. The practice of mindfulness (and the sitting meditation in particular, during which we observe our thoughts as simply thoughts) can be very helpful in becoming aware of this.

In the sitting meditation, we can recognize that thoughts come and go all the time. They are ephemeral and, in themselves, have no real substance. With patience and perseverance, we can experience this repeatedly in mindful meditation practice. In time, we will more easily recognize the transitory nature of stress-amplifying thoughts. Then, even in potentially difficult situations, we can let them flow by instead of giving them greater substance by trying to fight them off. If we can stay present without reacting while a chain of negative thoughts arises, it will grow ever easier to avoid entanglement in the net of associations that would otherwise ensnare us.

During an MBSR course, Sabine, a university employee, told us about her insomnia and how she managed to end the suffering it caused her:

> I have trouble falling asleep at night and often find myself lying awake for a long time. All kinds of thoughts and worries go through my head, and I feel wide awake. I used to try fighting it

off. I thought about how stressed I must be if I can't even get to sleep properly. I considered all sorts of solutions and got in a real state about how awful everything was.

Apart from that, my main problem was worrying about how on earth I'd manage to get up in the morning.

When I started practicing mindfulness, I realized I was aggravating the insomnia by trying to figure out what was causing it, by judging myself for it, and by blowing it up into an even bigger problem.

So now, when judgmental thoughts about my insomnia start up, I'm consciously aware of them and practice being mindful of my breathing instead of getting caught up in these negative chains of thought.

Now I can see it not as insomnia but as simply being awake, so I feel a lot calmer and more relaxed. More often than not I just fall asleep again; and if not, I'll just read a good book.

In any case it doesn't bother me anymore — instead of suffering, I just accept the fact that I'm awake.

How Our Relationship to Our Thoughts Can Shift

Some of our thought processes are extremely stubborn and tenacious, or perhaps so charged with emotion that we're too caught up to observe them objectively. Some thoughts are so powerful and so deeply embedded in the subconscious that we need to deal with them in other ways.

In these instances, cognitive strategies, such as questioning the content of the thoughts or making a reality check, can be very helpful. The first step to take when troublesome or distressing thoughts occur is to be consciously aware of the thoughts without trying to fight them off or criticize ourselves because they have surfaced (yet again). The idea is to cultivate an attitude of tolerance and self-acceptance, particularly in difficult situations. Then, if we notice that the thoughts are distressing, turbulent, and persistent, we can make a mindful decision to pause and ask certain questions about them (see box).

Helpful Questions to Ask Ourselves
in Relation to Recurring Difficult Thoughts

You may first acknowledge that difficult thoughts are present. Then, with friendliness and curiosity, ask yourself one or more of the following questions:

- Is this thought true? What proof is there?
- Will this thought actually help me achieve a result I desire?
- What would someone who wasn't in my situation think?
- How will I reflect on this situation later — tomorrow, or in a year?
- What is the worst that can happen? What exactly would be so terrible if it did happen?
- How likely is this worst-case scenario?
- Have I dealt with a similar situation in the past, and if so, how did I manage it?
- What would I tell a friend if he or she were in this situation?
- What would a good friend tell me about this situation?
- Is there anything that might help me feel more secure and courageous in this situation?

It can be very helpful to release feelings of guilt or shame, to tell yourself:

- I am allowed to make mistakes.
- I am allowed to not be able to do something.
- I am allowed to have weaknesses and to show them.

In situations that can't be changed, we can ask ourselves questions that inspire a shift in perspective:

- What can I learn from this situation?
- What meaning or understanding can I find in this situation?

Steps for Coping with Stressful Experiences through Mindfulness

- Consciously pause and feel your breath. This helps create a space between stress triggers and stress reactions so they do not happen automatically.
- Be aware of your body, and tune in to the early warning signs of stress.
- Be aware of potential stress-amplifying thoughts.
- Be mindful of your emotions.
- If necessary, make a conscious decision to do something else to help release the hold of stress-amplifying thoughts — for example, take a break or do an exercise or activity mindfully.

Welcoming All Emotions

Difficult or distressing emotions can also be stress triggers. Our thoughts generate and influence our emotions and vice versa. Emotions can reinforce our thoughts and make them seem more real. Our emotions help us recognize and identify our needs; and at the same time, they form the basis of decision-making processes in our everyday life.

In the sitting meditation learned in Week 5, we practice mindfulness of various phenomena, including the breath, the body as a whole, sensations, sounds, thoughts, and emotions. Practicing in this way allows us to recognize thoughts as thoughts and emotions as emotions. This is a vital step in working with the reactions to stress triggers, by slowly replacing automatic reactions with mindful responses. Automatic reactions do not run their course as easily as before, and we can be much more in touch with situations — and ourselves — as they unfold.

Emotions and Stress

Experiencing difficult or overwhelming emotions is one of the major factors in stress. For participants in MBSR courses, it is no different. Many people express interest in an MBSR program because they want to learn to be more skillful with their emotions. They express their concerns in various ways:

- "I'm often anxious, and that makes me feel stressed."
- "When I'm stressed out, I get angry and treat people unfairly."
- "I shout and yell and blame others, even when it's not their fault. This would have destroyed my marriage if it hadn't been for my wife's patience."

Some people experience their emotions by turning inward:

- "The greater the external stress, the more withdrawn and reclusive I become."
- "I'm not in touch with my feelings. In particular, I find it hard to vent my anger, which bothers me a lot. I've already suffered from a stomach ulcer."

Here are two very different ways of dealing with difficult emotions:

1. We suppress them until we aren't aware of them any longer, but they continue to have an effect on the subconscious.
2. We allow ourselves to be governed by our emotions, and they overwhelm us in stressful situations.

In both cases, we lose contact with our emotions and they tend to run us.

However, there is another option: by cultivating mindfulness and adopting a nonjudgmental attitude toward our emotions, we can learn to be with them openly as they occur. The more adept we become at recognizing and understanding our feelings, the better we can understand what we're experiencing emotionally at any given moment. We can be more in touch with what we need and how we can express that need — an important aspect of mindful communication.

Pausing and Becoming Aware of Our Feelings

In many spiritual traditions and schools of psychotherapy — from psychodynamic therapy to humanistic therapies like Gestalt — it is acknowledged that a natural and open approach to our feelings is an essential component of mental and physical health.

Feelings are part of our genetic makeup — they indicate our state of health and are crucial for survival. We "decide" on a very basic level, often before any sensory stimuli can even reach our thinking minds, whether we regard any given situation or event as pleasant, unpleasant, or neutral — the three basic emotional qualities of human experience, according to Buddhist psychology. Each quality triggers its own series of thoughts, feelings, and reactions. If we have a neutral experience, we don't give it a lot of attention — in other words, we don't ponder it for long — so our emotional reaction to a neutral event is indifference.

An unpleasant experience generates a reaction aimed at either minimizing, ending, or escaping from that experience, or suppressing memories (perhaps through denial or avoidance) of it while avoiding a repetition of the event. We start to analyze the situation, to question it, brood over it, and worry about it. We want to "get away from it," so our automatic response is a flight reaction accompanied by feelings ranging from fear, rejection, and denial to irritation, anger, rage, or guilt.

The opposite reaction is triggered when we have a pleasant experience — we want more. We seek to hold on to the experience, to magnify, extend, or repeat it, so we react with feelings of longing and attachment. This is the driving force behind many of our desires.

All of these reactions are perfectly natural and even have survival functions, since they help us gauge whether a situation is dangerous. In our everyday lives — particularly in our relationships with others and our feelings toward ourselves — we're rarely faced with life-or-death situations. Therefore it's important to recognize our emotional patterns clearly so that our lives are not controlled by them. This goes for avoidance behavior in particular. Avoidance is a survival instinct automatically triggered by an unpleasant experience. It can create problems and even lead to depression, chronic fear, or other psychological disturbances when it is used for coping with unpleasant emotions. Research by psychologist Steven Hayes has shown that the avoidance of unpleasant experiences or feelings (also known as experiential avoidance) lies at the heart of many emotional disorders, such as depression and anxiety disorders.

But if we become overattached to pleasant events, this can create problems too, since every experience passes with time, and clinging to its memory inevitably leads to suffering. Many of us know intuitively that trying to repeat a pleasant experience often leads to disappointment.

During the sixth week of the course, Elisabeth realized that she had been so thrilled with her experience of the body scan during Week 1 that she compared it to all her subsequent body scans. This is how she described her insight: "I was always waiting for that same wonderful physical sensation I had during my first body scan. But it was never that intense again, so I was a bit disappointed every time I practiced the body scan. I always thought I was doing something wrong, because it was never the same as the first time; I'm glad that I now know the reason why."

Our willingness to fully accept the reality of each moment as it is, is often conditional, and that goes for pleasant as well as unpleasant experiences. We strive to manipulate or control our reality. Mindfulness is about cultivating exactly the opposite attitude. And since dealing with our feelings in a natural, open manner is a much more helpful approach than avoidance, the practice of mindfulness is particularly helpful in supporting us so that we get in touch with our emotions as we develop a more relaxed attitude toward them.

Sitting meditation provides the ideal opportunity to practice being aware of our thoughts and emotions and thereby reinforces an attitude of pure observation. This helps us recognize that — just like sounds and physical sensations — our thoughts and feelings are ephemeral phenomena, which we can observe without having to change them. This is a challenging process, because we all tend to become enmeshed in our feelings and identify with them. Mindfulness helps us acknowledge, accept, or examine our emotions without being overwhelmed by them.

Locating Emotion in Our Bodies

With sustained mindfulness practice we can become increasingly aware of our feelings and develop the ability to distinguish between pleasant, unpleasant, and neutral experiences. The next step is to observe the chain of reactions that follows an experience: the thoughts and physical sensations that accompany them, as well as the feelings. By allowing an experience to occur by saying yes or hello to it, a bodily reaction can ensue — maybe our rib cage expands, or we find ourselves breathing more deeply, or we might notice a relaxed sensation in the abdomen.

If we say no to an experience, this may trigger other physical sensations: our stomach might contract, or we'll notice tension in our forehead, or we might clench our hands into fists. Our feelings invariably manifest themselves in physical reactions (which may be subtle or completely unconscious), and this is where mindfulness comes into play. Rather than pursuing a chain of thought — "I don't like this pressure in my stomach," for example — we stay with the physical sensation of pressure as much as we can. We can support ourselves by asking, "What sensations am I aware of?" Through mindfulness we can stay present with the physical sensations, rather than be carried away by thoughts about them.

I (Petra) once experienced firsthand how mindful awareness can transform difficult emotions, when I taught my first Mindfulness-Based Cognitive Therapy (MBCT) course. The course was part of a university research project, which meant I had to record the sessions on video and review them with the lead researcher at regular intervals. I had thoroughly prepared everything, and we had arranged to meet a few hours before the beginning of the first session. On my way to the meeting, I noticed that I was extremely nervous. My stomach was in knots, and my thoughts were all over the place. I obsessed over whether I had all the necessary documents and whether I'd prepared myself in every way possible. I went through the sequence of the lesson over and over again, and although I realized that I'd prepared and planned everything down to the very last detail, I couldn't shake off my anxiety. On the contrary, the closer I got to campus the more agitated I became. In the end, I developed a stomachache. This surprised me; I had never experienced such agitation before a seminar and had no idea what was causing it.

Initially I tried to hide my agitation from my colleague. After talking through various subjects, we decided to meditate together. During that meditation I tried to be mindful of the pressure in my stomach and to stay with it — which was not easy, since my thoughts kept trying to pull me away from that unpleasant sensation. But as I continued to meditate, I gradually became able to stay with the sensation and accept that it was there. At some point in the course of meditation, I realized that the massive pressure covered a deep fear: I was afraid of failing. My greatest fear was that my colleague would take one look at my videos and tell me it would be best if I never facilitated an MBCT course again. "You're just not cut out for this," I thought he would say.

The moment I expressed my fear, I immediately felt relief and my stomach relaxed. After the meditation, I shared my insight with my colleague, and this relieved the pressure in my stomach even more. Above all, mindfulness helped me realize how unrealistic my fear actually was. I was still a bit wound up, but it was nothing compared to the state I'd been in before. Once I'd recognized what was causing my fear, it lost its power to terrorize me. I was moved by the realization of how helpful it can be to stay with a body sensation without trying to change or analyze it. That evening I felt a great deal more in touch with myself than I had for some time.

Exercise: Mindful Awareness of the Body

The following exercise can help you be more aware of your body and physical sensations in daily life.

- Begin by sensing yourself in whatever position you are in: sitting, standing, lying down, or walking.
- Next, ask yourself: "What exactly am I experiencing in my body right now?" Allow yourself to open to any sensations that may or may not be present. Don't try to force, seek out, or produce any particular one. Just be aware of what is actually there right now, if anything. You need not change the experience in any way. Just stay with it as best you can from moment to moment. If you decide to change your posture, be aware of the sensation of movement in your body as you do so.
- You can also ask yourself: "What position are my arms in at the moment?" "What sensations do I have in my legs?" "Where are my legs in contact with the chair?" "How is my head positioned in relation to my upper body?" If you're walking, you may ask yourself: "What movements am I aware of?"
- From time to time, you may also become aware of sensations inside your body, such as a rumbling of the stomach, a throbbing or pulling feeling, pressure, or muscular tension. Be aware of the sensations outside your body as well.
- Explore practicing awareness of sensations on a regular basis during the day — whenever you think of it.

Ways to Be Skillful with Unpleasant Emotions

How can we become familiar with our feelings without being overrun by them or overidentifying with them? At the same time, how can we avoid repressing or denying those feelings?

Developing the ability to acknowledge our feelings, to know them for what they are and allow them to *just be* without fearing them, is a big step toward healing as well as being wholly aware of ourselves.

Every feeling is composed of a mixture of mental activity and physical sensations that often coalesces to form specific thoughts about the sensations. Through practicing mindfulness, we become increasingly aware that we cannot control thoughts and feelings that may arise. What we *can* do is make a conscious choice to be mindful of whatever surfaces. Here are a few steps you can take when encountering a difficult or unpleasant feeling:

- Pause, and be aware of your breathing.
- Become aware of any sensations in your body. Ask yourself: "Where exactly in my body is this sensation, and what do I feel there?" As best you can, stay with the sensation.
- Name the emotion present without identifying yourself with it. For example: "There is fear," "There is anger," "There is grief."
- Let this naming help you to feel and stay in contact with the emotion.
- Accept that the emotion is present: "Whatever it is, I allow myself to sense it."
- Continue to be present, as best you can, for whatever you experience.
- If this proves too difficult, you may return to awareness of breathing and, when you are ready, start again. Or you may decide to continue at another time.
- At the end of the meditation, ask yourself: "What do I need right now? What would be helpful for me right now?"

It's best to start by practicing with an emotion that is not too strong — for instance, a mild reluctance to tackle a particular task. Whenever you encounter this reluctance, pause and then become aware of the physical sensation accompanying the emotion. Be as kind to yourself as possible. In the next step, try to express the emotion in words. For example: "I feel reluctance. I accept this reluctance right now. It is okay for me to feel this way." Stay with the emotion for a few moments, and when you are ready, ask yourself if it has changed in any way and, if so, how.

You may also want to devote a few minutes of your sitting meditation practice expressly to mindful awareness and acknowledgment of emotions over a certain period. In Week 5, participants practice daily mindful awareness of their sensations and emotions, both during the formal sitting meditation practice and in everyday life.

Once we become fully aware of and acknowledge our emotions, we can express them in a skillful way and communicate them to others. We explore this in the next weekly session of the MBSR program.

Mindful Communication

The greatest gift we can give others is the gift of our own presence.
When we listen mindfully, without judgment, we gift our listeners with
*   trust and openness.*
And we support them so that they can express themselves mindfully.

— Linda Lehrhaupt

The sixth session begins with a sitting meditation. After spending some time checking in about the students' home practice, we turn to the main theme of this session: mindful communication. Exercises presented in class allow a direct experience of mindful communication in action. Two that we frequently use are as follows:

1. Students pair off, and one person describes a problem he or she recently experienced (we ask people to keep it simple, and we suggest examples like getting stuck in traffic or something breaking at home), and then the listener repeats what he or she heard. This is followed by the speaker expressing whether she or he felt understood. Then the speaker and listener switch roles.

2. In a role-playing exercise, participants experiment with and observe different styles of communication classified as passive, aggressive, or mindful.

Through these and other exercises, we experience the rich exchange of mindful communication.[26]

Communication: A Major Cause of Stress

MBSR class participants often report that difficulties in communication are one of the most frequent causes of stress in their lives. Why, then, do we wait until more than halfway through the course to introduce a topic that causes difficulty for almost everyone? What do we mean by difficult or stressful communication?

In the following cases, all four people describe a situation in which they experienced a difficult communication:

Mary, a fifty-two-year-old accountant, noted, "I don't feel heard by my husband. I have explained to him repeatedly that I cannot sit by and watch him ruin his health by smoking sixty cigarettes a day and overeating. I know it's been hard on him since he was laid off, but it's hard on me as well. I've had to take on extra work, and I don't have time at home with the kids anymore. No matter how often I tell him, he just doesn't listen."

John, a thirty-eight-year-old garage owner, said, "I don't know what to do anymore. The pain from the car accident last year is terrible. I've told my partner that I need more time off, that I have to take longer breaks, and that sometimes I can't come in at all. I asked my doctor to increase the dosage of pain medication, but he refused. Both of them seem to think that because I'm up and about, there's no real problem. Nobody seems to give a damn!"

Peter, a seventy-three-year-old retired teacher, told us, "My wife is losing more of her memory every day. I have tried my best to take care of her, but it's getting beyond my capability. She sometimes gets lost or forgets to turn off the gas. I mentioned to my daughter that maybe we should look for a home for her, but she just flew into a rage and accused me of all sorts of things. I love my wife. How could my daughter say those things to me?"

Sabine, a twenty-two-year-old student, said, "I don't want to go on with my studies. It was a mistake in the first place. I chose medicine only because my father wanted me to. But I really want to travel, study languages, and maybe teach in other countries. My parents have said they will cut me off if I don't finish school. Every day, it's getting worse for me. I'm even thinking of flunking some of my exams to get out of this mess."

Each of these MBSR class participants had the same theme: they didn't feel listened to. Moreover, because of that, they felt angry, frustrated, helpless, overwhelmed, lonely, or unsupported. They also shared an underlying assumption: if people would listen to them, those individuals would act to fulfill the speakers' wishes. For example:

- Mary's husband would stop smoking and take better care of himself.
- John's partner would encourage him to take time off.
- Peter's daughter would not accuse him of abandoning her mother and would maybe even help him find a nursing home for her.
- Sabine's parents would allow her to drop her medical studies and take time off.

The Focus of Mindful Communication: Ourselves

Mary, John, Peter, and Sabine each focused on the hope that someone else would give them what they wanted — attention, validation, or understanding.

This wish is understandable and very human, but articulating such a wish creates pressure on the listener. And when people feel that level of pressure from others, they tend to close up rather than open. Many feel threatened, resentful, and not heard, and this colors their responses.

In MBSR, rather than turning the spotlight on the person we wish to communicate with, we focus on how we ourselves behave in a situation of difficult communication. Participants tune in to their own thoughts, emotions, and physical sensations and observe them. By being aware of these, we gain important clues that can help us stay more balanced and centered. This in turn encourages us to be more mindful rather than reactive in our responses. In other words, we connect with ourselves first, before we try to connect with others.

In the previous weeks of the course, we have practiced being aware of sensations, emotions, and thoughts while doing the body scan, yoga, and sitting meditation. This mindful awareness can also be applied in times of difficult communication. By this point in the course, many participants have also developed the ability to recognize the difference between being mindfully in touch with their needs or wishes and being lost in or absorbed by them.

Mindful communication as we practice it in MBSR embodies careful and sensitive attention to how we express ourselves. This expression is shaped by principles of deep listening, respect, and openness to different points of view. We cannot know how another person will react, and we cannot control how someone will behave. However, we can do our very best to take care of ourselves and try to interact with others in a way that embodies mutual regard, clarity, and responsibility.

Sometimes participants have the misunderstanding that to communicate mindfully means to be passive or silent. They feel confused because they think engaging in mindful communication means they should not speak out against injustices or abusive behavior. Others think that practicing mindful communication means we cannot make requests of others or ask something for ourselves.

The late Dr. Ulla Franken, a member of our institute faculty and an expert on the role of emotions in healing and health care, spoke of how being in touch with our emotions and learning to express ourselves in a clear, nonblaming way is an essential aspect of mindful communication.

> When communicating with others, it's often hard to express exactly what we want or don't want. We've probably all hidden behind a statement such as "We really ought to..." (go to the movies, do sports together, or maybe clean up the kitchen), instead of saying what we want: "I'd like to have fun with you," or "I could do with a nap: Would you mind doing the dishes?"

Sometimes — particularly when we are angry or upset — we tend to blame others and complain about their behavior. It's often easier to criticize someone else ("You're always late"; "You never make an effort") instead of staying with our own experience and feelings.

A mindful approach can make a big difference to the course of the conversation. Take, for example, the difference between saying "You are inconsiderate" and "I feel ignored." In the first case we are shifting the blame onto the other person and putting them on the defensive. In the second example, we are taking our fair share of the responsibility, giving the other person more room to maneuver.

Embodying a mindful approach to communication is very different from passivity, silence, or helplessness. Indeed it is a vibrant form of communication that supports clarity, forthrightness, and humane action.[27]

Journal of Difficult Communication

In preparation for the class on mindful communication, participants are asked to keep a daily journal.[28] Once a day for one week, they each describe an instance of difficult communication by answering questions about it. They are asked to explain the situation, who was involved, what the MBSR student wanted from the situation, and what the other person(s) seemed to want. They are also asked to describe how they felt during and after the situation. Finally, they are asked if the problem was solved. During Week 6, we invite participants to share entries from their journals either in pairs or in the larger group.

Klaus's journal entry about an incident with his son exemplifies how learning to practice mindful communication can have a profound effect on a person's assessment of a situation. Klaus, a fifty-two-year-old businessperson who had survived two major heart attacks, told his classmates:

The situation of difficult communication involved my son. He's twenty-three years old and still living at home while he attends college. I had asked him to buy groceries on his way home from school. I was going to cook my special dish that I knew everyone liked. It was the first time in weeks that the whole family would be able to have dinner together....

When I got home and wanted to start cooking, I saw he had not shopped for the things I asked for. He was in his room with the music blasting. I knocked on his door, and when he opened it I asked him about the shopping. "Sorry, Dad," he said, "I forgot." And then he shut the door in my face. I could feel the blood rush to my head. My heart started pounding, my breathing increased rapidly, and I felt tightness in my chest. The thought flashed through my mind — "Calm down, it's not worth another heart attack."

I backed away from the door and my hand went to my heart. I tried to calm down by focusing on my breathing. My son opened the door, took one look at me, and came rushing toward me. "Dad, are you all right?" he asked anxiously. "Do you need your medicine? Should I call an ambulance?"

I looked into his face and saw fear in his eyes. All of a sudden, my anger was gone. I found myself saying, "I'm okay now. But I am disappointed. I wanted to cook the special meal you all like."

My son looked at his watch and said, "Dad, the stores are still open. I got caught up with this difficult project and I just forgot. I've got the list right here. I'll be right back." And before I could say anything, he was out the door.

Klaus looked down at his journal entry, then continued:

I have to admit, these questions in the book really helped me understand something. I got so angry because I thought my son completely ignored me...but it wasn't it at all. In the past I would have yelled all sorts of things at him. How he was a no-good, living off his mother and me. Not taking responsibility. Just shooting out my anger. Instead, I stuck to telling him how I felt. It was hard...it's a big shift for me. But it sure beats having another heart attack.

Key Aspects of Mindful Communication

Be in Touch with Yourself

Using Klaus's story, we can look in more detail at some key aspects of mindful communication. First, Klaus tuned in to his own physical sensations: he became aware of his racing pulse, red face, and tight chest. He recognized that these sensations were a warning that he was in an agitated state. For a man with a history of heart trouble, this is not a good place to be.

It is doubtful that Klaus would have been able to stay with his own feelings and physical reactions had he not been practicing mindfulness in the weeks leading up to this incident. By his own admission, he tended to lash out without thinking when he felt hurt or threatened.

His awareness of his own physical sensations in this stressful situation helped break a cycle of escalation that had been usual for him in the past. In stepping away from the door and tuning in to himself, he reminded himself to focus on the here and now rather than get lost in habitual reactions.

Be Present

As Klaus stood with his hand on his chest, a thought came to him: "It's not worth another heart attack." In not reacting in the usual way, and staying in the present moment, a new possibility arose for him. In this more open and less reactive space, Klaus became aware that preventing a heart attack was his top priority. This reminded him that he needed to take care of himself first.

Make Contact with the Other Person

By not reacting and instead taking a step back, Klaus was able to rest in a more open space that allowed him to connect with his son. Because Klaus did not attack the young man the moment he opened the door, his son was not on the defensive as he might have been had his father yelled at him. Klaus saw that his son indeed cared about him; he was able to note the fear in his eyes. Rather than be blinded by his own anger, Klaus recognized the deep love and concern that his son felt for him.

Express Your Needs by Using "I Messages"

When Klaus expressed his hurt feelings, he said it was hard — and new — for him. He did the best he could. In the past, he might have said to his son, "You're a disappointment!" Instead, he used an "I message" and said, "I am disappointed."

By saying how he felt, Klaus was practicing a key aspect of mindful communication: expressing his own needs or his take on a situation by using "I messages." These are statements that describe how we feel emotionally at the moment, by using the pronoun *I* and referring to ourselves. They express how we perceive a situation from our individual perspectives. "I messages" are nonaggressive and nonblaming. They express the speaker's personal experience instead of generalizing and insisting that the speaker's own feelings are the whole story.

In the case of Klaus, he was able to say he felt disappointed without recrimination or anger.

Suggestions for Using "I Messages"

1. Speak about yourself, about your own feelings and thoughts. Focus on your own experience and allow it to unfold. Inform others as much as possible about what the experience represents for you.
2. Focus on any wishes you have in relation to the other person, and express them as best you can. Discuss together how your wishes could be met in a way helpful to you and respectful of the other.
3. Let the other person tell you what she or he understood from your communication and how she or he experienced your words.
4. Avoid declarations about what the other person is thinking or feeling. These often prompt others to feel defensive and close down.   — Ulla Franken

Perhaps it is clearer now why the theme of mindful communication is first introduced in the sixth week of an MBSR course. As we have seen, the communication exercises draw on mindfulness skills that have been practiced from the beginning of the course: staying connected with ourselves and turning inward. Without mindfulness, we would be prone to react rather than pause, to project blame or anger onto someone else, or to withdraw into a sense of helplessness.

By not reacting, blaming, or withdrawing, we allow the space to stay open in the situation. Mindfulness practice supports us so that we remain present, calm, and steady. This is in sharp contrast to the tension that can dominate a situation fueled by reaction, anger, panic, or blame.

This open space supports deep listening, which is listening beyond assumptions, definitions, or undeclared needs. As we practice deep listening — to ourselves and to others — we build connection and community.

A Day of Mindfulness: Deepening the Practice in Stillness

Silence is the element in which great things fashion themselves together.

— Thomas Carlyle

A full day of mindfulness practice takes place between the sixth and seventh sessions of an MBSR course. Taking place in silence, this day offers a unique opportunity to maintain the continuity of mindfulness practice over an extended period. Many experience this day as an intensification of their mindfulness practice.

Being silent in a group can be challenging and, at the same time, a wonderful experience. Many people especially value the opportunity to be silent, and they may say something like: "I don't need to talk today. I can be in contact with people without feeling forced to speak."

In everyday life, we often feel obliged to communicate. When we are with someone, we think it would be rude not to engage in conversation. But on this retreat day, everyone remains silent together, thus making it easier not to talk, even if it might initially feel disconcerting. Practicing in silence means that we create an inner space where we can be with ourselves and find the way to our own hearts.

During the day, we refrain from conversation or other forms of communication — gestures, facial expressions, eye contact, or smiles.

This gives participants the space to be fully with their own pleasant, unpleasant, or neutral emotions as we practice mindfulness while sitting, walking, lying down, or standing. We eat a communal lunch in silence, too, which permits everyone to eat with the same mindful awareness experienced in the raisin exercise during Week 1.

Silence helps our minds to rest. Just as sand stirred in a tumbler of water gradually settles to the bottom and leaves the water clear if we let it rest for a while, so the agitation of our minds and stressful thoughts can gradually settle as well. Our minds generally become calmer, clearer, and more open. During the Day of Mindfulness, many participants experience a sense of inner peace they have seldom known before.

The introduction at the opening of the day allows participants sufficient opportunity to raise any questions or voice any concerns before the day starts. At a sharing period at the end of the day, people have a chance to talk about their experience of the retreat. Often people express how their fears or preconceptions have shifted. Many participants say something like: "Only now do I understand what practicing mindfulness really means."

The teacher announces during the introduction that anyone can speak to him or her during the day, if necessary. In our experience, this happens rarely; but it's important that the option exists, because the silence is intended to be supportive rather than oppressive.

All the mindfulness exercises we've learned so far (body scan, yoga, and sitting meditation) are practiced during the retreat. We add one new exercise (if it has not already been introduced), and that is walking meditation (see box on page 152). In the afternoon after lunch there are exercises in movement and in stillness, followed by a guided meditation. The final activity is a mindful group sharing, after the teacher breaks the silence by asking participants to speak softly to each other in pairs. The day ends with a short sitting period. Most participants feel enriched when they go home. We often hear people say things like these:

"I feel so happy and fulfilled — I'm quite proud of myself."

"I never thought I could hold out in silence for all that time. I found that not only could I bear it, but I also really got a lot out of it."

"It wasn't easy, and I got a bit bored sometimes, but now I feel fantastic. I'm glad I had this experience, and it's good to know I can live without talking all the time."

Walking Meditation

It is the quiet paths, not the major highways, that lead to the heart.

— Turkish proverb

There are many different paths of mindfulness, one of which is the practice of walking meditation. During walking meditation we direct our full attention to each step we take, being mindful of the physical sensations. To begin with, it's helpful to practice walking meditation as a formal mindfulness exercise (see box on page 152). In everyday life it is also possible to integrate elements of walking meditation into daily activities, such as taking a stroll in the park.

Choose a place where you can take about fifteen or twenty steps without any obstacles. This could be at home or outside. It helps to walk slowly at first so you can more easily be aware of each part of the walking movement. The rhythmic pace of walking helps slow down mental activity and calms the mind. At times when the mind is particularly restless and our thoughts are racing, walking meditation may be more practicable than sitting meditation. While the body is in motion, our minds focus on a specific activity — namely, the act of walking — and this helps the flood of thoughts to gradually slow down.

There are many different types of walking meditation. Here, we describe the type we practice as part of our MBSR courses.

Exercise: Walking Meditation

- Start by deciding on the amount of time you want to devote to a session of walking meditation — for example, ten or fifteen minutes.
- To begin, stand still for a moment at your starting point and become aware of your body in the standing posture. You may want to allow your arms to hang loosely by your sides; or if you prefer, you can bring them together and clasp them in front of your midriff or behind your back. Allow your shoulders to relax downward.
- If you like, you can close your eyes for a moment while bringing your awareness fully to your body.
- You may also leave your eyes open and gaze downward about a yard's distance in front of you. Feel the distribution of weight on your feet and the sensations in your legs, your back, the front of your body, your arms, shoulders, and head. Don't try to change any of these sensations; we practice simply being aware of them.
- When you are ready, open your eyes if they are closed and start walking forward slowly.
- With every step you take, be aware as best you can of the sensations of movement. You may be aware of the pressure of your foot on the ground, the lifting of your foot, the shifting of your weight from one foot to another. Just take one step…and another…and another…and another!
- Once you reach the end of the distance you set for yourself, pause for a moment and be aware of your body. Then turn around slowly, pause again for some moments in the standing posture, and walk back along the same route. Continue walking back and forth in the

same way, remaining aware of your sensations and of the process of walking.

- If you find your mind wandering (which will happen during walking meditation, as it does during any other meditation), just be aware of it in a gentle and nonjudgmental way. Then turn your attention to the step you are in the process of taking and any sensations present. Continue the walking meditation until you reach the end of the time period you established in the beginning.
- As you end the walking meditation, stand for a few moments in stillness, sensing your whole body. Then bring the meditation to a close in whatever way you find most comfortable.

WEEK 7 · Taking Care of Ourselves

Participants arrive for the class in Week 7 after having taken part in the Day of Mindfulness a few days before. They have spent a whole day together in silence, practicing mindfulness meditation and eating lunch in stillness. While the class has already spent six weeks together, the feeling of community, reinforced by the Day of Mindfulness — the sense of being on the path together — deepens. A number of our class participants have told us how moved they were when they looked around the room at the beginning of Week 7 and knew they had done a silent retreat together. Many of them had felt concern before the day (Can I make it? Will it be too hard?). Now there is a quiet sense of accomplishment and commitment. Not for everyone, of course, but for many.

In Week 7, various exercises are introduced under the general theme of exploring how we take care of ourselves. And implicit — and explicit — in this exploration is the idea that mindfulness, through both formal and informal practice, can be intentionally harnessed in the service of self-care. In Week 7, and continuing in Week 8, the focus is also on how mindfulness practice can be integrated into everyday life. Not merely theoretically, but in practical and down-to-earth ways that will allow all to carry the practice forward into their lives once the class is over.

After a short period of sitting, the group practices standing yoga exercises. To begin with, a short body scan while standing may be introduced. Because they have practiced the body scan in the weeks before, class members are invited to notice what is present. They are also invited to notice whether any parts of their bodies are asking for care: maybe they feel tension in their shoulders from working at the computer, or their eyes are tired from too much reading. They simply tune in gently to their bodies during the scan, noticing any sensations that may be calling for their kind attention.

Then they may be asked to share what they noticed in their bodies, as well as whether there is a standing yoga posture — or perhaps another exercise (like rolling the shoulders) — that they would like to do now and share with the group. Perhaps it has become a favorite posture, or they are enacting an intuitive understanding that, "when I am feeling a certain way, I can do this yoga pose to express my wish to take care of myself." Many have experienced over the preceding weeks a more natural ease in their yoga postures as well as a gentleness that spills over into how they move in everyday life.

As someone leads the exercise, he or she can comment on it at the same time, sharing a personal relationship to it. The stories participants tell in this context are not always rosy, but they are true. Invariably, some say that it was only through doing yoga that they realized how much they had ignored themselves or treated themselves harshly.

One participant, a former marathon runner, shared the following: "I was so angry that I could not get my foot to sit right up at the top of my leg during the standing pose. Since my hip operation, it's impossible. No matter what I do, I can't get anywhere near where I used to." He paused a moment before continuing. "I pushed so hard I fell over one time. I was lucky. But my pride took a beating. But as I look at all of you, I can feel something else: You see, we're all standing tall, and we're standing proud." And he added with a smile: "Even if most of us are a bit crooked."

An important aspect of self-care is recognizing that the most important factor in actually doing it is our own willingness to "step up."

So often, especially if we have experienced an assortment of difficult setbacks, we can become passive or unengaged, waiting for someone or something else to engage us. Stepping up to self-care is really about accepting the invitation from our own body, mind, and heart to reconnect again and again, to listen carefully, to become aware of whatever messages are being sent, and responding appropriately. Noting that our shoulders are tight and stretching them is responding to the same kind of impulse that reminds us to take our medicine or go for a long-overdue checkup or speak with someone about a conflict. *Self-care* means taking care of the self. And since one of the most difficult things for many of us is not only recognizing when we need care but also giving it to ourselves, an exercise such as this one is profoundly self-nourishing.

The next exercise explores the theme "Wherever you go, there you are," a wise saying that is also the title of a bestselling book on mindfulness meditation by Jon Kabat-Zinn. Guided in silence throughout the exercise by the MBSR teacher, class participants are invited to move to different seats in the room according to a particular set of themes that are explored at each "seating." The exercise also calls attention to an important quality that is strengthened by mindfulness: the capacity to exercise choice. Touching on this subject at various times during the course, we explore how mindfulness can help us make wise choices by being aware of habitual behavior and the mind-set that keeps us locked in and locked up.

Participants are invited to explore the direct sense of where they are, and the attitudes they have about being there, as they move to different places in the room that they choose for their seemingly unpleasant or pleasant experiences. At each seat they may ask themselves questions suggested by the teacher. Some of the questions point to the expectations someone may have about his or her experience. For example, at one point participants are invited to sit in a place they assume is unpleasant, a place they might normally never have chosen. Tuning in to their sensations as they sit in the seat, becoming aware of the different experiences they take in through their senses, many are pleasantly surprised that their actual experience is other than what they thought it would be. Perhaps they see things from a completely different perspective that is afforded by the new position. For example, someone may have often felt cold in the room, but the new sitting place is in a sheltered corner and there is protection from a draft.

At the same time, a place chosen for its assumed pleasantness can also be unpleasant because the seat does not allow someone to sit comfortably, or sitting there makes the participant feel closed off from the rest of the room. So the exercise allows a participant to practice being with whatever is present, whether it is pleasant, unpleasant, or neutral.

The fact is, most of the time we are not where we are. We may be wishing to be somewhere else, or we may be so caught up in our own opinion that we see not what is there but only what we are conditioned to see. As a result, our world becomes smaller and smaller because we tend to confine ourselves to what we know, even when we are not particularly happy there. Is it possible to see beyond or within what we perceive, to take off our blinders and be willing to be with what is, as it is?

The teachers will probe the relationship between the exercise and its application to everyday life, perhaps asking, "Do you see a connection between this exercise and the theme of expectations in your own life?" Or: "Which seat do you take in your life?" Or: "If things are unclear or uncertain, can you allow for not knowing?"

The theme of the ever-changing nature of things and situations also comes up, and once again the practice of mindfulness — understood as our being with whatever arises, wherever we are — is underlined. Even the uncertainty has a right to be there. Being reactive means wanting to get rid of discomfort as soon as possible. Being responsive means allowing the situation to unfold by staying with it from moment to moment. And in the unfolding, a new sense of calm and stability can take root, even when everything around us is tossing and turning.

The fear of not being in control often stops us from entering a new situation where we face the unknown. For some, the idea of exploring new places can appear to be attractive. But for the person who strongly resists the unfamiliar, it is anything but comforting. I (Linda) know this very well from my own experience. I visited Paris at least three times before I allowed myself to settle in and enjoy the city. Even though I was born and raised in New York City, I was extremely uncomfortable the first few times I went to Paris. Each time I left after one day and went to a smaller French city or town. It was only when I was invited to stay with someone in Paris that I felt comfortable enough to explore the city.

As I reflect back, making allowances for being quite young and quite broke when facing Paris's challenges, I recognize that it was mostly my sense of not knowing where I was, of having lost control, and of not being able to negotiate my way around well enough that caused me to flee. I felt helpless because I could not speak the language; and since I was not good at map reading, I often ended up somewhere other than where I wanted to be. I wanted to skip over the insecure phase of the unfamiliar as quickly as possible, and I literally checked out of Paris before I ever checked in.

Martina shared an experience with a similar theme. She had been struggling to get away as quickly as possible from discomfort, but it was impossible for her because the source of her "private hell," as she termed it, was literally in her head. Severe tinnitus had prompted her to enroll in an MBSR course. She had been receiving both medical treatment and psychotherapy, but so far neither had produced the effect she had hoped for. She had been skeptical about whether the course would help her, but she wanted to give it a try. Most difficult for her so far had been the sitting meditation:

> I thought I would jump out of my skin the first time the teacher asked us to listen to sounds. I had been doing everything I could not to listen to sounds, because those inside my head were driving me crazy. I couldn't escape. But I managed to keep going, although, for a long time, all I could feel was my resistance, sometimes tears, and lots of pressure...inside and out. At some point, though, I stopped fighting, stopped trying to keep the sounds at bay. I accepted them...I mean, I accepted that they were there. And it was a revelation! I saw (heard) things about them I never had before. They were not all the same, and there were even small moments when they were not there at all. I don't know what

happened, but I became aware of something for the first time: I can live with them!

Following the place-changing exercise, a period of extended sitting meditation takes place, deepening the experience of sitting in the midst of our lives through the practice of open awareness. Because this exercise follows the movement exercise, it reminds participants that they have indeed taken their seat, and that it is possible to be present in the middle of their lives. Choiceless awareness, which they began to practice in Week 5, is more familiar now, and the instruction to be with what is — to be present for sounds, the breath, thoughts, emotions, and sensations — feels familiar.

After sitting meditation, time is taken to explore the home practice. Now in Week 7, the group is more often self-guiding, relying less on guidance from the teacher. Group members may ask each other questions or for more details about a point made. They experience more trust and clarity and engage in a deeper level of exploration. Wisdom emerges naturally in the group.

The next theme we explore is: "What do I take in?" As part of their home practice, participants have reflected on this theme during Week 6. The following is some guidance for your home practice and is based on an MBSR course workbook for class participants from the Institute for Mindfulness in Rolde, the Netherlands.[29]

Noticing What You Take In

Each day we take in a great deal through our five senses: sight, hearing, touch, smell, and taste. The senses are entrances to our awareness and can give rise to automatic reactions: we find an experience either pleasant or unpleasant, and the next thing we do may be to decide that we really want this or really don't want that.

This week, give particular attention each day to what you are taking in through the senses. Notice what you hear, see, smell, feel, and taste, and consider the following:

- Where does it come from?
- How much of it do you take in?

- Does it happen more or less automatically, or is it a conscious choice?
- Is it neutral, pleasant, or unpleasant?
- How does your body react to it? And your breath?
- What feelings or thoughts are present?
- What do you notice about the way you are with it?

In class, participants are invited to share what they noticed during the week before class. While they mention many things, the three most often discussed are food, digital media, and noise. Eating comes up for many during the week. Many comment on being aware of the difficulty of staying with the experience as it happens. They mention various forms of what they call mindless eating, including:

- eating on the go
- eating quickly in order to get it out of the way
- eating while completely engaged in another activity
- making unhealthy food choices
- overeating when stressed

At this point, it is easy to slip into focusing on how-to solutions or to assume that there is a right and a wrong way. Particularly difficult is our tendency to beat ourselves up as a way of trying to force ourselves to be the way we think we should be.

The emphasis in this class session is on noticing, sensing, and becoming aware of how our bodies and minds are affected by cravings. The point is not to provide solutions or tips. In fact, both observation and research studies have shown that such approaches do not have a long-lasting effect on changing behavior. Finding the capacity to ride the sensations that prompt us to engage in a particular behavior, and yet not doing so, can be far more helpful. One reason is that what we feel is a response, rather than a reaction, and it is self-nurturing rather than self-punishing. By cultivating a gentle and quiet resolve, rather than judging ourselves, we create a foundation of self-trust and a sense of quiet mastery that tells us: "I can do this. Even when I backslide, I can notice it without jumping on myself and can just move forward again. Again and again..."

Reactions do occur, and in class we strongly emphasize noticing that the reaction manifests from a decentered position. We can choose to see thoughts as thoughts rather than as a drive to do something. Often participants wish not to react, and although they may be aware of this, it does not always lead to healthier choices, since habits are deeply ingrained. We may find that we criticize ourselves at this point, but self-compassion and trust are called for. One important question that arises in class is: How can we maintain our awareness in daily life?

The effects of living in an increasingly digital world come under scrutiny for many participants as they observe what they take in, or what they expose themselves to, during the week. They also worry about the amount of time they spend on the internet, especially on social media, and how it is affecting their family or other social relationships.

The effects of social media are clearly apparent in public life. Many people constantly consult their devices. In restaurants we often see whole families consulting their smartphones while seated at tables, barely taking time to order. According to Jeanene Swanson, "There's also the trend of not being able to live in the moment — without broadcasting every detail in text, tweet, or social media share. It speaks to a larger issue, in internet-speak FOMO, also known as the dreaded Fear Of Missing Out."[30] She cites David Greenfield, founder of the Center for Internet and Technology Addiction in Connecticut, who comments on an effect of "living" online: "I can't say it's a pathology but it's an interesting social phenomenon," Greenfield says. The problem becomes: "you're not really living [life], you're transmitting it."[31]

What role can mindfulness play in helping us live a truly balanced life, where neither food nor internet usage nor any other substance or activity takes up too much of our lives and leaves us insufficient time for nourishing activity and periods of rest? The latter two are necessary if we are to keep our stress levels low and cultivate resilience and the capacity to wind down after a stress challenge.

One key aptitude that we address especially in Week 7, but also in the weeks before, is the capacity to notice when we are involved with something that is not helpful to us. By noticing it, we interrupt the automatic tendency to move toward engaging in the behavior. Moments like these are in fact opportunities where choice becomes possible. The times when we experience an increased awareness of these moments, even if only briefly, are powerful indicators — and possibilities — for participants.

Further, the practice of mindfulness allows us to be aware of how quickly and harshly we judge ourselves, inadvertently strengthening our sense of being out of control or victims of our own impulses. There is a strong tendency, when confronted with habitual behavior, to feel negative about it and to want to fix or change it as quickly as possible. This is another example of a reactive response, which is fueled by the wish to get rid of something we don't like. Another way to describe this is to say that we feel aversion toward something; it causes discomfort, which we want to relieve.

To wish to change is a human quality, but perhaps the most helpful place to begin is not by trying to make any changes at all but by cultivating the capacity to pay close attention to when this wish appears and to the way it affects us. We can pay attention on a bodily level, noticing our sensations, thoughts, and emotions and their effect on us. We can resist the urge to make our response stop and instead ride the waves of impulse, paying close attention to where they manifest in our body.

We could say that we are mindfully hanging out in the space between impulse and the movement toward satisfaction. It is not an easy place to be, but with practice and the cultivation of curiosity and kindness rather than self-punishing and critical attitudes, we water the seeds of wisdom that may one day flower into wise and life-giving choices.

In an earlier part of this book we talked about the willingness to simply be with a habit of avoidance, rather than adopting the sense that we have to be disciplined and overcome something. We talked about the experience of Robert, who felt he did not have the discipline to continue to practice every day during the MBSR course. The word *discipline* is often used in the context of changing unhealthy life choices. We say we are undisciplined if we cannot avoid taking that extra piece of chocolate, and yet the harsh drive to be disciplined, which is considered a form of self-improvement, is in fact an act of aggression toward ourselves. Rather than using the word *discipline*, which often connotes punishing or unkind behavior, Linda prefers the word *willingness*.[32] Willingness, in this context, is the quality of being present, in body, mind, and heart, in an open awareness without grasping at, shutting down, or amplifying what is there. Another word that could be substituted for *discipline* is *wholeheartedness*.

Pema Chödrön, whose books have been bestsellers because of their warm and practical approach, has this to say about the path of wholeheartedness:

> Wholeheartedness is a precious gift, but no one can actually give it to you. You have to find the path that has heart and then walk it impeccably. In doing that, you again and again encounter your own uptightness, your own headaches, your own falling flat on your face. But in wholeheartedly practicing and wholeheartedly following that path, this inconvenience is not an obstacle. It's simply a certain texture of life, a certain energy of life. Not only that, sometimes when you just get flying and it all feels so good and you think, "This is it, this is the path that has heart," you suddenly fall flat on your face. Everybody's looking at you. You say to yourself, "What happened to that path that had heart? This feels like the path of mud in the face." Since you are wholeheartedly committed to the warrior's journey, it pricks you, it pokes you. It's like someone laughing in your ear, challenging you to figure out what to do when you don't know what to do. It humbles you. It opens your heart.[33]

So practicing with a spirit of wholeheartedness is in fact the act of returning again and again to a situation, with kindness and determination as our skillful partners.

As the class draws to a close, we call attention to the fact that the next class is the final one. In the workbook on home practice, class members are asked to reflect on their aims for continuing practice once the course is over. How will they keep up the momentum they have generated in the preceding weeks? Wholeheartedness, kindness, and leaning into life are seeds that have been planted and watered, and that can be harvested, moment by moment, again and again. In the moments of stillness that conclude the class, participants embody a sense of quiet confidence, soft determination, and mindfully being present right here, right now.

Questions to Support Mindfulness
When Confronting Impulse, Craving, and Aversion

When you notice a craving or impulse to do something you would normally engage in, try asking yourself one or more of the following questions. It's best to see each question as an open space in which you can simply be present with whatever comes up, rather than as an item on a to-do list that you have to check off.

1. First notice: What is drawing you to engage in the activity? What do you seem to want really badly?
2. Take time to note:
   a. What sensations are present? Where are they located in your body?
   b. Are thoughts present (e.g., "I've got to have this" or "I've got to relieve this pressure")?
   c. Are any feelings present (e.g., sadness, restlessness, anger, joy)?
   d. How can you be mindful while experiencing a desire to either reach for something or try to avoid it?
   e. Do you really want something, or is there something unpleasant you want to cover up or block?
   f. Is there something else that would in fact be healthier and more satisfying for you?
   g. How would whatever you are pulled toward influence your health or feeling of well-being?
   h. What alternatives might be possible?
   i. What obstacles seem to prevent you from choosing a healthy alternative?

Looking Backward, Going Forward

The last session of an eight-week MBSR course begins like the previous ones: with a mindfulness exercise. Starting with the body scan, the group comes full circle, repeating an exercise introduced in the first session. By now the body scan is familiar, as are the yoga postures and the sitting and walking meditations. In addition, each of the exercises is, as before, an invitation to come home to ourselves.

The MBSR Course as a Journey

In many ways, taking part in an MBSR course is similar to going on a journey. As is true when planning a trip, there are many things to take care of: registering for the course, arranging for transportation, adjusting schedules, and so on. Before a trip begins, we usually acquire maps and guidebooks. If we study them long enough, we might think we know what to expect. However, a trip will often provide surprises for which no book could have prepared us.

It is the same with reading anything (including this book) about the MBSR program before experiencing it. No matter how much information we absorb, it soon becomes apparent that attending class is quite different from reading about it. As the semanticist Alfred Korzybski famously stated, "A map is not the territory it represents."

During a trip, we often meet new people and sometimes travel with them before going off in separate directions. There is often a sweet sadness at parting. A similar feeling pervades the last session of an MBSR course. Even if the journey together has not always been smooth, there is a spirit of camaraderie and a sense of having traveled on the path of mindfulness together. Acknowledging this during the last meeting of the group is poignant for many. During the eight weeks, however, they have practiced allowing such feelings to be present without either encouraging them or pushing them away.

Becoming Our Own Best Friend

A theme we take up in the last session is how to continue mindfulness practice once the course is over. For many participants, signing up for the MBSR class was an important step in this direction. As the course ends, we take time to reflect on what we have learned about caring for ourselves and how we can continue to do this in the future.

One of the ways we do this is to ask participants during Week 7 to reflect on the following questions and to pick one or more that seem to be particularly relevant:

- Which activities support my health, personal growth, and relationships? Which activities seem to harm these areas of my life?
- Can I make time in my daily life to engage in a physical exercise that I enjoy on a regular basis?
- What do I need to do to put my ideas for taking care of myself into action?
- What and who can sabotage my plans? What concrete steps can I take to support myself if hindrances appear?
- Is it possible to reach out to another person? How can I do that? Perhaps by:

  1. exchanging phone numbers with someone and speaking together on a regular basis as meditation coaching partners?
  2. enrolling in a graduate MBSR course or other mindfulness meditation offerings?

3. going on a retreat?

4. meditating with a friend or group on a regular basis?

Sometimes participants are invited to write a letter to themselves and seal it in a self-addressed envelope that their teacher will send to them several months later. They are encouraged to use words of support for themselves in the letter, especially about continuing their mindfulness practice in the future. They are also encouraged to remind themselves of what they learned during the course.

Many participants are deeply moved when they read their letters months later. Helen wrote to tell of her experience:

> When I first received the letter, I couldn't believe I wrote those words. They sounded so wise. Was it really me? And when I read them again, I knew it was indeed me who had written them.
>
> The MBSR course helped me connect to the deepest part of myself, a part that knew then, and will always know, how I should take care of myself. I reread the letter every so often to help me stay on track. After all, I am reading a letter from my very best friend.

The Eternal Flame: Keeping the Practice Going

At the end of the course, many participants ask themselves: How will I continue my mindfulness practice when the weekly class is over?

Before the Olympic Games begin, a torch is lit in the stadium. The flame is a powerful symbol of the spirit of dedication, commitment, and training that enables the event to happen every four years. The first session of an MBSR course is much like lighting a flame that symbolizes the spirit of mindfulness. Each time we practice an exercise, we are fanning the flame, encouraging it to burn bright.

It was not always easy to keep the flame burning during the course. Sometimes a strong wind or rain threatened to extinguish it. The inclement weather could have been anything, from something simple to profoundly life-altering: the alarm clock failing to go off, a last-minute project at work that could not wait, or a loved one rushed to the hospital.

Life happened. Wonderful, crazy, peaceful, challenging, and sometimes hurricane-strength events took place. Meeting life and staying present in the middle of it, neither running away nor falling apart, was our practice. Now, how do we keep going?

Going Straight on a Road That Has Ninety-Nine Curves

Hans expressed his concern about continuing his mindfulness practice after the course was over: "I worked hard these eight weeks to establish a regular practice. I am afraid that once there is no class to come to, I will not be able to keep it up. There was something really helpful about knowing I was coming here every week. And now that will fall away."

No one says that it is easy to practice mindfulness in daily life, and especially not when difficulties arise, whether this means severe pain, unemployment, a personal tragedy, or being buffeted by life's unpredictability. What many discover during the course, however, is that mindfulness is empowering. Learning that it is possible to be aware of the various aspects of a difficult situation, and becoming able to make a conscious decision about how to respond, nurture both a sense of personal strength and a desire to make a responsible choice.

Sabine confirmed this when she said on the last evening of her course: "How do I keep up the practice, even though it feels like life gets 'in the way?'" She laughed, looked around at her classmates, and continued. "Well, life doesn't get in the way, does it? Life happens. The real question is: How do I respond to it?"

Sabine's statement points to a central theme of mindfulness practice: How do we keep going in the face of difficulty? Indeed, this is a central theme in many meditation traditions. In the practice of Zen meditation, for example, students sometimes engage in a form of meditative inquiry where they reflect on stories that appear at first to be paradoxical. The question of how to keep going in the face of difficulty in life is similar to a well-known Zen meditative question: How do you go straight on a road that has ninety-nine curves?

When students work with this question, their first reaction is usually: "But that's impossible. You can't go straight on a road with ninety-nine curves." After reflection, however, a student may see that the road with ninety-nine curves is her or his own life. The curves are events that happen every day: setbacks, challenges, and opportunities.

If we think we have to go straight on the winding road, it could mean we think that we have to plow through life without looking left or right. However, going straight could also mean that we accept life's invitation to meet it directly: by going straight on and turning into every curve as best we can — not blindly, but allowing ourselves to stay open to what we meet along the way. We learn to trust our own capacity to live a mindful life and experience its richness no matter what the circumstances.

Continuing Formal and Informal Practice

In preparation for the final session, participants are encouraged to design their own schedules for their practice once the course is over. Some decide to focus on one of the formal exercises and practice that regularly. Others prefer a mixture — for example, dividing their sixty minutes of daily practice time into segments in which they do either the body scan or yoga, followed by a period of sitting meditation.

Participants are also encouraged to experiment, during Week 7, with doing the main meditation exercises without audio guidance. The message is that we all have everything we need to integrate mindfulness into our lives on a daily basis, and that we can take a stronger role in deciding what our mindfulness practice will look like and how we will structure it in terms of our available time.

For many it is clear: mindfulness practice has to be a priority in their daily lives. Joan shared with us her experience about making practice a priority:

I had an appointment last week that was very important to me. It was pouring rain that day, and I didn't have a car. I decided to call a taxi, but I was worried there would be none available. So I called a taxi three hours before I needed it to make a reservation. I even told a little lie and said I had to go to the doctor.

I amazed myself at the effort I made. It was a great lesson to me about putting commitment behind a decision. I saw that I could do the same thing with my mindfulness practice. I just have to set it up, commit to it, and, rain or shine, just do it. It's really up to me, in the end.

Radical Honesty

To be realistic about continuing mindfulness practice is to make plans based on knowing yourself and designing a practice in daily life that is doable.

It makes no sense to say that you will get up every morning an hour earlier than usual to practice, if you know you are not a morning person or you have very young children whose waking time can be unpredictable. Reflecting on the following questions can be helpful in setting up a realistic practice plan:

1. What has been possible for me to do in the past?
2. Ideally, how would I like to schedule my mindfulness practice for the future?
3. Is this plan realistic?
4. What hindrances may arise?
5. What resources can I draw on to help me?
6. What further adjustments are necessary to make my plan as viable as possible?
7. Can I commit to this? For how long?

We encourage you to take your time with these questions and your answers. You might have to tweak them a bit. For example, perhaps you decide not to practice on Mondays because it is normally a difficult day for you. Continue to shape your plans until you find something you can commit to...and then commit to it!

Often, a natural question arises: What happens if I stop practicing? The training in mindfulness is no different than training in other skills. If you learn a musical instrument as a child, for example, and then stop for a time, you may still be able to play years later. But you will miss more of the notes, your hands will feel much stiffer, and the music may feel strained because you have not practiced on a regular basis. If you begin to practice again, it will take some time but agility will return.

The same is true whenever we stop mindfulness practice. We can always begin again...and again...in the next moment...with the next breath.

Working with the question of how to maintain our practice requires us to be radically honest. *Radical* in this sense means that we are willing to observe our own behavior and name it for what it is. It means seeing clearly, and not only through the veil of our hopes, wishes, and expectations. Then, when we don't meet our goals, we pick ourselves up as kindly and gently as possible, dust ourselves off, and start all over again. It is powerful to name things for what they are, quietly and courageously decide what needs to be done, and then do our best.

The End Is the Beginning

As the final class moves toward its close, each person has an opportunity to say what was important for him or her in the course. To introduce this theme, Linda sometimes reads the following true story from the book *Presence* to her students:

> Several years ago...Fred told a story that moved people very deeply. A few years earlier he had been diagnosed with a terminal disease. After consulting a number of doctors, who all confirmed the diagnosis, he went through what everyone does in that situation. For weeks he denied it. But gradually, with the help of friends, he came to grips with the fact that he was only going to

live a few more months. "Then something amazing happened," he said. "I simply stopped doing everything that wasn't essential, that didn't matter. I started working on projects with kids that I'd always wanted to do. I stopped arguing with my mother. When someone cut me off in traffic or something happened that would have upset me in the past, I didn't get upset. I just didn't have the time to waste on any of that."

Near the end of this period, Fred began a wonderful new relationship with a woman who thought that he should get more opinions about his condition. He consulted some doctors in the States …and soon after got a phone call saying, "We have a different diagnosis." The doctors told him he had a rare form of a very curable disease. And then came the part of the story I'll never forget.

Fred said, "When I heard this over the telephone, I cried like a baby — because I was afraid my life would go back to the way it used to be."[34]

Many course participants are inspired by Fred's story and are eager to share how mindfulness has affected, shaped, and imprinted their own lives.

As the class ends, everyday life, as always, is waiting. As she did every week before, Sarah waves good-bye and rushes to catch the last bus. John's phone rings as soon as he turns it on; his wife asks him to pick up milk on the way home. Mary helps Jane with her coat. Allan stands behind Jane's wheelchair, ready to roll her down to the entrance, where her husband is waiting with the van. Carl calls out to Fred, "Send me the reference for the article. Maybe there is something there for me."

Final good-byes are said, the classroom empties, and soon a quietness settles in the once busy space. Life continues elsewhere, everywhere. Next week the class will fill with participants for the new course. The cycle will start all over again.

In the week to come, Sarah, John, Allan, Mary, Jane, Carl, and Fred will open their workbooks to read the entry for home practice following the last session. They will find these lines from a letter written by the poet Rainer Maria Rilke in his book *Letters to a Young Poet*:

> I beg you...to have patience with everything unresolved in your heart and to try to love *the questions themselves* as if they were locked rooms or books written in a very foreign language. Don't search for the answers, which could not be given to you now, because you would not be able to live them. And the point is, to live everything. *Live* the questions now. Perhaps then, someday far in the future, you will gradually, without even noticing it, live your way into the answer.[35]

May these words guide us all with patience and wonder on the road of ninety-nine curves.

Acknowledgments

We would like to start by thanking the founders and pioneers of MBSR. Their commitment in passing the teachings on to the next generations, as well as their dedication in encouraging or carrying out related research, has proved to be of immeasurable value, not least to the authors of this book.

In particular, we express our appreciation to Jon Kabat-Zinn, the founder of MBSR and an extraordinary teacher and visionary. His unstinting commitment and foresight paved the way for MBSR to thrive worldwide. We also thank Saki Santorelli, who continues a tradition of excellence as executive director of the Center for Mindfulness in Medicine, Health Care, and Society, at the University of Massachusetts Medical School. Our deep thanks also go to Florence Meleo-Meyer, director of the Train-the-Trainer Program, Oasis Institute for Mindfulness-Based Professional Education and Training at the Center for Mindfulness (CFM), who with gentle wisdom and warmth has shared generously with us and all who have studied with her. Furthermore, we thank Melissa Blacker, Elana Rosenbaum, and Ferris Urbanowski, with whom we have trained, and who provided inspiration and clarity and shared their love of teaching MBSR.

We also express our heartfelt gratitude to Mark Williams, one of the founders of Mindfulness-Based Cognitive Therapy, for his support and sound advice as well as his inspired way of teaching. Many thanks also to Rebecca Crane, director of the Centre for Mindfulness Research and Practice at Bangor University, Wales, for her wise counsel and skillfull teaching, as well as her commitment to the development and dissemination of criteria for assessing teachers of mindfulness-based interventions. We were also greatly enriched by our relationship with Paul Fulton, a member of the faculty of the Institute for Meditation and Psychotherapy and all our colleagues in this field. The following colleagues and friends read the manuscript and made helpful suggestions: Cornelius von Collande, Christoph Egger-Büssing, Ulla Franken, Thomas Heidenreich, Karin Krudup, Renee Kraemmer, Jörg Meibert, Christa Spannbauer, and Ingrid van den Hout. We are grateful to them for their help in making the book as accessible, accurate, and useful as possible.

We are grateful to New World Library for their enthusiastic support in publishing the English version of our very successful German edition, and to Jason Gardner, our editor, and Bonita Hurd, our copyeditor.

We also thank the editor of our German edition, Heike Mayer, for her skillful editing, helpful feedback, and continued support. In an early stage of the English-language version of this book, we were supported by our editor Alice Peck and copyeditor Linda Carbone.

A special thanks to Norbert Wehner, who not only read the manuscript carefully but also spent many hours incorporating editing changes into the text.

Our appreciation also extends to our colleagues Nils Altner, Bernd Langohr, Katharina Meinhard, and Ulla Franken, who kindly gave us permission to use some of their texts and ideas. Furthermore, we thank members of the IMA faculty, especially Sagra Hannich, Günter Hudasch, Karin Krudup, Malgosia Jakubczak, Frits Koster, Johan Tinge, Maureen Treanor, Erik van den Brink, and Ingrid van den Hout, who have graciously been available for consultation and who offered wise support. It's a privilege to work with such an inspiring, imaginative, and creative team of teachers and researchers.

A very special thanks to the heart of the Institute for Mindfulness-Based Approaches — the core office staff and coordinators — who work in such a dedicated and committed fashion. Many, many bows of gratitude to Thomas Schaaff, Hildegard Evels-Schaaff, Susanne Schneider, and Sylke Känner. Former office staff who contributed significantly to the development of the institute deserve a heartfelt mention: Michaela Diers, Silke Kraayvanger, and Irene Leupi.

Linda wishes also to express her deep gratitude to Sabine Stückmann, who in 1997 provided inspirational and practical support to enable her to participate in the first Teacher Development Intensive of the Center for Mindfulness, Worcester, Massachusetts. Sabine was then a young woman with a vision, and Linda has done her best to honor her request to help MBSR flourish, first in Germany and later throughout Europe.

Linda also offers warm thanks to Peggy Hunter and Dave Tate, who in 1995 allowed her to do an internship in their MBSR classes at LDS Hospital in Salt Lake City, Utah. In these relatively early days of MBSR in the United States, they made an important contribution to establishing MBSR in hospital settings.

We were touched by the openness and willingness of participants in the various programs in which we have taught to share and learn together. In many respects, they were our teachers, gifting us with their clear eyes and warm hearts.

We also express our deep appreciation to our meditation teachers. Linda Lehrhaupt bows to Al Fusho Rapport, Sensei, who has guided her with wisdom, compassion, and humor. She is also grateful to Genpo Merzel, Roshi, and Nico Tydeman, Sensei, with whom she studied for many years.

Petra Meibert is deeply indebted to her first teacher, Don Alexander, for making the practice of mindfulness accessible in a way that helped her integrate it into her life and open up to the path of meditation. Additionally, she expresses her profound gratitude to her teacher Tarab Tulku Rinpoche and his patient and knowledgeable support on the path of practice.

Petra Meibert expresses her deepest feelings of connectedness and gratitude to her husband, Jörg, for his loving support and encouragement during the writing of this book. Thank you for your professional and constructive criticism, for providing emotional support whenever obstacles appeared, and for giving me the courage to carry on.

Linda Lehrhaupt expresses her unbounded appreciation to her daughter, Taya, and to her husband, Norbert. Thank you, Taya, for supporting me in tough moments and encouraging me to trust myself and do what needed to be done, even when it was not easy. Norbert, your support in the form of loving encouragement, your capacity to cut through to what is essential, and the wonderful meals you have cooked up at the drop of a hat have nourished me on all levels. Thank you for always being there, come what may.

Notes

1. Jon Kabat-Zinn, *Full Catastrophe Living: Using the Wisdom of Your Body and Mind to Face Stress, Pain, and Illness* (New York: Bantam, 2013), p. xxxv.
2. Ibid., p. lxii.
3. An excellent source for up-to-date information on research into mindfulness is the *Mindfulness Research Monthly,* published by the American Mindfulness Research Association, https://goamra.org/publications/mindfulness-research-monthly.
4. The Center for Mindfulness in Medicine, Health Care, and Society at the University of Massachusetts Medical School has offered MBSR since 1979 to more than twenty-two thousand people at the Stress Reduction Clinic. Europe has seen strong growth in the teaching of MBSR, where today there are many hundreds of teachers, in Germany, the Netherlands, Switzerland, and the United Kingdom. Other European countries in which we know MBSR is being offered include Denmark, Finland, France, Greece, Ireland, Italy, Lithuania, Norway, Poland, Spain, Sweden, and Turkey. MBSR is also being taught in Argentina, Australia, Brazil, Hong Kong, New Zealand, Peru, South Africa, South Korea, Taiwan, and other countries around the world. In the United States, the Center for Mindfulness in Medicine, Health Care, and Society has organized a conference each year on MBSR and related interventions. The German MBSR-MBCT Teachers Association also organizes a conference each year that attracts hundreds of participants from German-speaking countries. A European umbrella association of MBSR teachers associations known as the European Network of Associations of Mindfulness-Based Approaches (EAMBA) brings together teachers across Europe for meetings and retreats. In fact, some national health services in European countries (for example,

in Germany) are offering reimbursements to their insured clients when they participate in an MBSR course.

5. Kabat-Zinn, *Full Catastrophe Living*, p. 268.

6. P. Grossman, L. Kappos, H. Gensicke, M. D'Souza, D. C. Mohr, I. K. Penner, and C. Steiner, "MS Quality of Life, Depression, and Fatigue Improve after Mindfulness Training," *Neurology* 75, no. 13 (2010), 1141–49.

7. Richard Davidson and Sharon Begley, *The Emotional Life of Your Brain: How Its Unique Patterns Affect the Way You Think, Feel, and Live and How You Can Change Them* (New York: Penguin, 2012), p. 11.

8. Ibid., p. 205.

9. Ibid., p. 204.

10. Kabat-Zinn, *Full Catastrophe Living*, pp. xli–xlv.

11. Lucia McBee, *Mindfulness-Based Elder Care: A CAM Model for Frail Elders and Their Caregivers* (New York: Springer, 2008).

12. Kabat-Zinn, *Full Catastrophe Living*, p. xlii, xlix.

13. Darlene Cohen, *Turning Suffering Inside Out: A Zen Approach to Living with Physical and Emotional Pain* (Boulder, CO: Shambhala, 2002).

14. "365 Days of Happiness," *Daily Good*, undated, www.dailygood.org/2010 /07/20/365-days-of-happiness.

15. Zindel V. Segal, J. Mark G. Williams, and John D. Teasdale, *Mindfulness-Based Cognitive Therapy for Depression: A New Approach to Preventing Relapse* (New York: Guilford Press, 2002), p. 184.

16. Charlotte J. Beck, *Everyday Zen* (San Francisco: HarperCollins, 1997), p. 140.

17. Stephen Levine, *Meetings at the Edge: Dialogues with the Grieving and the Dying, the Healing and the Healed* (New York: Anchor, 1984), p. 133.

18. "Perlman Makes His Music the Hard Way," *Houston Chronicle*, February 10, 2001, www.chron.com/life/houston-belief/article/Perlman-makes-his-music -the-hard-way-2009719.php; "Three Strings and You're Out," Snopes.com, last updated May 16, 2007, www.snopes.com/music/artists/perlman.asp.

19. "If I Had My Life to Live Over — I'd Pick More Daisies," www.devpsy.org /nonscience/daisies.html. This story, too, probably belongs to the urban legends genre. In any case, the story gets told over and over again and seems to have inspired many people.

20. Segal, Williams, and Teasdale, *Mindfulness-Based Cognitive Therapy for Depression*, p. 170.

21. Nils Altner, extract from *Manual for MBSR Course Instructors*, Linda Lehrhaupt & Karin Krudup, eds. (Bedburg: Institute for Mindfulness-Based Approaches, 2016), p. 75. This manual is not available outside our training program.

22. Ibid. A different version can be found in German in Nils Altner, *Achtsam mit Kindern Leben: Wie wir uns die Freude am Lernen erhalten; Ein Entdeck-ungsbuch* (Munich: Kösel, 2009), pp. 87–88.

23. Katharina Meinhard, extract from *Manual for MBSR Course Instructors* (Germany: Institute for Mindfulness-Based Approaches, 2009), p. 108. This manual is not available outside our training program.

24. Shinzen Young, "Pure Experience," *Buddhadharma* (Spring 2007): 38.

25. Richard S. Lazarus and Susan Folkman, *Stress, Appraisal, and Coping* (New York: Springer, 1984).

26. The exercises that we use for our mindful communication classes draw on those of the MBSR curriculum developed by Jon Kabat-Zinn and staff members at the Center for Mindfulness. Another exercise that we sometimes use during the communication session was developed by Dr. Edel Maex, a Belgian MBSR teacher.

27. Ulla Franken, extract from *Workbook for MBSR Course Participants* (Bedburg: Institute for Mindfulness-Based Approaches, 2016), p. 43. This workbook is not available outside our training program.

28. The daily journal for stressful communication can be found in Kabat-Zinn, *Full Catastrophe Living*, appendix, pp. 614–15.

29. From *MBSR Course Participant Handbook of the Institute for Mindfulness*, ed. Johan Tinge, et al. (Rolde, Netherlands: Institute for Mindfulness, 2016).

30. Jeanene Swanson, "The Neurological Basis for Digital Addiction," The Fix, October 6, 2014, www.thefix.com/content/digital-addictions-are-real-addictions.

31. Ibid.

32. Linda is inspired to use the word *willingness* by the definition of the word *discipline* by Zen teacher Charlotte Joko Beck, as "the willingness to look again and again at what is."

33. Pema Chödrön, *The Wisdom of No Escape* (Boston: Shambhala, 2010), p. 96.

34. Peter Senge, C. Otto Scharmer, Joseph Jaworski, and Betty Sue Flowers, *Presence: Exploring Profound Change in People, Organizations and Society* (London: Nicholas Brealey Publishing, 2005), pp. 25–26.

35. Rainer Maria Rilke, from *Letters to a Young Poet*, Stephen Mitchell, Trans. Boston: Shambhala, 1993), pp. 49–50.

Recommended Reading

Please note that the books on our list are intended primarily for the general public. We have also narrowed our list to focus mainly on MBSR but have included a few books on other mindfulness-based interventions as well.

Bardacke, Nancy. *Mindful Birthing: Training the Mind, Body, and Heart for Childbirth and Beyond*. San Francisco: HarperCollins, 2012.

Bartley, Trish. *Mindfulness-Based Cognitive Therapy for Cancer*. Oxford, UK: Wiley-Blackwell, 2012.

Bates, Tony. *Coming through Depression*. Dublin: Gill and Macmillan, 2011.

Bauer-Wu, Susan. *Leaves Falling Gently: Living Fully with Serious and Life-Limiting Illness through Mindfulness, Compassion and Connectedness*. Oakland, CA: New Harbinger, 2011.

Bays, Jan Chozen. *How to Train a Wild Elephant: And Other Adventures in Mindfulness*. Boston: Shambhala, 2011.

———. *Mindful Eating: A Guide to Rediscovering a Healthy and Joyful Relationship with Food*. Boston: Shambhala, 2009.

Biegel, Gina. *The Stress Reduction Workbook for Teens: Mindfulness Skills to Help You Deal with Stress*. Oakland, CA: New Harbinger, 2009.

Bowen, Sarah, Neha Chawla, and G. Alan Marlatt. *Mindfulness-Based Relapse Prevention for Addictive Behaviors: A Clinician's Guide*. New York: Guilford, 2011.

Brach, Tara. *Radical Acceptance: Embracing Your Life with the Heart of a Buddha*. New York: Bantam, 2003.

Brantley, Jeffrey. *Calming Your Anxious Mind: How Mindfulness and Compassion Can Free You from Anxiety, Fear and Panic*. Oakland, CA: New Harbinger, 2003.

Burch, Vidyamala, and Danny Penman. *Mindfulness for Health: A Practical Guide to Relieving Pain, Reducing Stress and Restoring Wellbeing*. London: Piatkus, 2013.

Carlson, Linda, and Michael Speca. *Mindfulness-Based Cancer Recovery: A Step-by-Step MBSR Approach to Help You Cope with Treatment and Reclaim Your Life*. Oakland, CA: New Harbinger, 2011.

Chödrön, Pema. *When Things Fall Apart: Heart Advice for Difficult Times*. Boston: Shambhala, 1997.

Davidson, Richard, with Sharon Begley. *The Emotional Life of Your Brain: How Its Unique Patterns Affect the Way You Think, Feel, and Live — and How You Can Change Them*. New York, Penguin, 2012.

Flowers, Steve. *The Mindful Path through Shyness: How Mindfulness and Compassion Can Free You from Social Anxiety, Fear and Avoidance*. Oakland, CA: New Harbinger, 2009.

Gardner-Nix, Jackie. *The Mindfulness Solution to Pain: Step-by-Step Techniques for Chronic Pain Management*. Oakland, CA: New Harbinger, 2009.

Germer, Christopher. *The Mindful Path to Self-Compassion: Freeing Yourself from Destructive Thoughts and Emotions*. New York: Guilford, 2009.

Hanh, Thich Nhat. *The Miracle of Mindfulness: An Introduction to the Practice of Meditation*. Boston: Beacon Press, 1999.

Hanh, Thich Nhat and Lilian Cheung. *Savor: Mindful Eating, Mindful Life*. New York: HarperCollins, 2010.

Kabat-Zinn, Jon. *Coming to Our Senses: Healing Ourselves and the World Through Mindfulness*. New York: Hyperion, 2005.

———. *Full Catastrophe Living: Using the Wisdom of Your Body and Mind to Face Stress, Pain, and Illness*. Rev. ed. New York: Bantam, 2013.

———. *Wherever You Go, There You Are: Mindfulness Meditation in Everyday Life*. New York: Hyperion, 2005.

Kabat-Zinn, Myla, and Jon Kabat-Zinn. *Everyday Blessings: The Inner Work of Mindful Parenting*. New York: Hachette, 1998.

Kaiser-Greenland, Susan. *The Mindful Child: How to Help Your Kids Manage Stress and Become Happier, Kinder and More Compassionate*. New York: Free Press, 2010.

Koster, Frits, and Erik van den Brink. *Mindfulness-Based Compassionate Living: A New Training Programme to Deepen Mindfulness with Heartfulness*. London: Routledge, 2015.

Lehrhaupt, Linda. *Tai Chi as a Path of Wisdom*. Boston: Shambhala, 2001.

McBee, Lucia. *Mindfulness-Based Elder Care: A CAM Model for Frail Elders and Their Caregivers*. New York: Springer, 2008.

Neff, Kristen. *Self-Compassion: The Proven Power of Being Kind to Yourself*. William Morrow: New York, 2015.

Rosenbaum, Elana. *Being Well (Even When You're Sick): Mindfulness Practices for People with Cancer and Other Serious Illnesses*. Boston: Shambhala, 2012.

Saltzman, Amy. *A Still Quiet Place: A Mindfulness Program for Teaching Children and Adolescents to Ease Stress and Difficult Emotions*. Oakland, CA: New Harbinger, 2014.

Santorelli, Saki. *Heal Thy Self: Lessons on Mindfulness in Medicine*. New York: Bell Tower, 1999.

Shapiro, Shauna, and Linda Carlson. *The Art and Science of Mindfulness: Integrating Mindfulness into Psychology and the Helping Professions*. Washington, DC: American Psychological Association, 2009.

Silverton, Sarah. *The Mindfulness Breakthrough: The Revolutionary Approach in Dealing with Stress, Anxiety and Depression*. London: Watkins, 2012.

Snel, Eline. *Sitting Still Like a Frog: Mindfulness for Kids and Their Parents*. Boston: Shambhala, 2013.

Stahl, Bob, and Elisha Goldstein. *A Mindfulness-Based Stress Reduction Workbook*. Oakland, CA: New Harbinger, 2010.

Stahl, Bob, Florence Meleo-Meyer, and Lynn Koerbel. *A Mindfulness-Based Stress Reduction Workbook for Anxiety*. Oakland, CA: New Harbinger, 2014.

Teasdale, John, Mark Williams, and Zindel V. Segal. *The Mindful Way Workbook: An 8-Week Program to Free Yourself from Depression and Emotional Distress*. New York: Guilford, 2014.

Williams, Mark, and Danny Penman. *Mindfulness: A Practical Guide to Finding Peace in a Frantic World*. London: Little, Brown, 2011.

Williams, Mark, John Teasdale, Zindel V. Segal, and Jon Kabat-Zinn. *The Mindful Way through Depression: Freeing Yourself from Chronic Unhappiness*. New York: Guilford, 2007.

Resources

Research

Mindfulness Research Monthly

https://goamra.org/publications/mindfulness-research-monthly

For an up-to-date listing of research about mindfulness-based approaches, please consult this valuable resource. It is also possible to subscribe to periodic updates.

Mindfulness-Based Teacher Project

A Podcast Series by Linda Lehrhaupt, PhD

In the *Mindfulness-Based Teacher Project*, Dr. Linda Lehrhaupt has created a forum in which to share her more than thirty-five years of experience as a teacher of mindfulness-based approaches. She brings her rich and extensive experience to an inspiring and down-to-earth podcast series designed to support teachers in the fields of mindfulness-based interventions, mindfulness in various contexts, mindful movement, and contemplative traditions.

The intention behind this motivational and informative series is to explore themes that touch the inner lives of teachers, as well as to help them deepen their teaching skills. At the same time, many others who don't teach mindfulness find the podcasts personally and professionally helpful.

Please visit www.mindfulness-based-teacher-project.org, where podcasts can be downloaded at no cost. They are also available free of charge on iTunes, SoundCloud, and Facebook.

The beautiful illustrations for each podcast are drawn by the artist Norbert Wehner.

Finding an MBSR Teacher

The number of MBSR teachers around the world is growing all the time. And the number of countries where MBSR is being taught is also increasing rapidly. We can list only a few resources here that may help you find a teacher. While the list is not comprehensive, we hope it will aid you in getting started.

You can also search the internet in your own country by typing in "MBSR" and then the geographic location in which you are interested in finding a teacher.

Please note: We provide the following information about MBSR teachers and organizations as a service, but in doing so we are not specifically endorsing or recommending any of these organizations or teachers. Please verify for yourself the teachers' qualifications and offerings to see if they are suitable for you.

MBSR Teachers Trained by the Institute for Mindfulness-Based Approaches

On the English- and German-language websites of the Institute for Mindfulness-Based Approaches, you will find a listing of IMA-certified teachers, from at least fifteen European countries, who have been trained by the IMA and who offer MBSR courses. Please check the IMA website from time to time for updated listings, because countries and teachers are continually being added to the list.

English-language website: www.institute-for-mindfulness.org/mbsr /Find-an-MBSR-teacher-near-you

German-language website: www.institut-fuer-achtsamkeit.de/mbsr/mbsr-lehrende-finden

North America

UNITED STATES

The following is a small sampling of the institutions and individuals who offer MBSR courses and/or various teacher-training initiatives. Many more opportunities to learn MBSR in North America are available than we have listed here. To find others, please search the internet in your area.

Center for Mindfulness in Medicine, Health Care, and Society, University of Massachusetts Medical School, Worcester, MA

www.umassmed.edu/cfm.

Founded by Jon Kabat-Zinn, the center is a pioneer in the development and teaching of MBSR. It also trains MBSR teachers throughout the world and has been a beacon and a model for quality and integrity in the teaching of mindfulness-based approaches.

CFM Certified Teachers in North America (and around the world)

The CFM has created a registry of teachers certified by them. Please see www.umassmed.edu/CFMInstructorSearch/app/#/index/search.

Duke University Integrative Medicine, Durham, NC

www.dukeintegrativemedicine.org/programs-training/public/mindfulness-based-stress-reduction

InsightLA

www.insightla.org/mindfulness/mbsr

Mindfulness Meditation New York Collaborative

www.mindfulnessmeditationnyc.com

Mindfulness Northwest, Pacific Northwest

www.mindfulnessnorthwest.com

Awareness and Relaxation Training,
Santa Clara and Santa Cruz Counties, CA

www.mindfulnessprograms.com

Mindfulness Institute of the Jefferson Myrna Brind Center
of Integrative Medicine, Philadelphia

http://hospitals.jefferson.edu/departments-and-services
/mindfulness-institute

Osher Center for Integrative Medicine, San Francisco

www.osher.ucsf.edu/classes-and-lectures/meditation-and-mindfulness
/mindfulness-based-stress-reduction

University of California San Diego Center for Mindfulness

https://health.ucsd.edu/specialties/mindfulness/programs/mbsr

CANADA
There are many MBSR offerings in Canada. Here are some that we are
aware of. Please do an internet search for yourself to find additional
offerings close to you.

MBSR British Columbia

www.mbsrbc.ca

Canadian Mental Health Association, Manitoba and Winnipeg

http://mbwpg.cmha.ca/programs-services/courses/mindfulness
-based-stress-reduction

Centre for Mindfulness Studies, Toronto

The center offers MBCT and other mindfulness-based approaches and interventions.
www.mindfulnessstudies.com/about/faculty

MBSR Ottawa

http://mbsrottawa.com

Meditation for Health, Toronto

www.meditationforhealth.com

Mindfulness Everyday, Toronto

www.mindfulnesseveryday.org

Mindfulness Institute.ca., Edmonton

www.mindfulnessinstitute.ca

Compassion Project, Winnipeg, Manitoba

www.chcm-ccsm.ca/compassion-project

Europe

THE EUROPEAN NETWORK OF ASSOCIATIONS OF
MINDFULNESS-BASED APPROACHES (EAMBA)

This is a European umbrella organization for teachers associations that was set up to facilitate dialogue and collaboration between institutions and representative bodies of teachers of MBSR and MBCT across Europe.

On EAMBA's website you will find a list of member organizations in various European countries. The websites of these national groups often list teachers within individual countries.

See http://eamba.net

MBSR Teacher Associations and/or Course Possibilities,
Listed by Country

The following list includes sources for finding an MBSR teacher outside the United States and Canada. They include national associations
of MBSR teachers, many of whom list MBSR teachers in their countries.

Both the IMA website (www.institute-for-mindfulness.org) and the
Center for Mindfulness website (www.umassmed.edu/cfm) offer international lists of teachers. In some cases we have listed individual
teachers who have trained with the Institute for Mindfulness-Based
Approaches or the Center for Mindfulness in Medicine, Health Care,
and Society. In other cases, we have included teachers we are familiar
with or have worked with. Some of them teach in countries that do
not have associations: others are members of listed associations, but we
wanted to list them individually nevertheless.

There are surely other teachers or organizations that we are not
aware of, and so we encourage you to do an internet search for yourself.

Argentina	www.mindfulness-salud.org
Australia	www.mtia.org.au
	www.openground.com.au
	www.alisonkeane.com.au
	www.mindfulnesstnsa.com
	www.simplymindful.com.au
	www.mindfulnesstnsa.com
Austria	www.institut-fuer-achtsamkeit.de/mbsr/mbsr
	-lehrendende-finden
	www.mbsr-verband.at
	www.mbsr-mbct.at
Belgium	www.mindfulmoment.be
	www.aandacht.be
	www.levenindemaalstroom.be
China	kevin.fong.gt@gmail.com

Czech Republic	www.lessstress.cz
	www.mbsr.cz
	www.praveted.info/MBSR
Denmark	www.mindfulness.au.dk
	www.mindfulness-mbsr.dk
Finland	www.mindfulness.fi
France	www.association-mindfulness.org
	www.euthymia.fr
	www.mind-ki.eu
Germany	www.mbsr-verband.de
	www.institute-for-mindfulness.org/mbsr/Find
	-an-MBSR-teacher-near-you
Greece	www.mindfulness360.net
Hong Kong	s.helen.ma@hkcfm.hk
	www.petamcauley.com
	junechiul@yahoo.com.hk
	www.mindfulnesshk.com
Hungary	www.mbsr.hu
Ireland	www.institute-for-mindfulness.org/mbsr
	/Find-an-MBSR-teacher-near-you
	www.themindfulspace.ie
	www.sanctuary.ie
	www.mindfulness.ie
	www.cfmi.ie
	www.ucd.ie
Israel	www.mbsrisrael.org
	www.mindfulness.co.il
Italy	www.mindfulnessitalia.it
	www.meditare.org
	alexandra.hupp@eui.eu
Korea	www.mbsrkorea.net
Lithuania	julius.neverauskas@neuromedicina.lt
	www.psichoterapija.info
	giedre.zalyte@gmail.com

Luxembourg	www.organisationen-beraten.net
	www.einfach-hier-und-jetz.de
	www.mbsr-trier.de
Mexico	www.mindfulness.org.mx
Monaco	kenya1955@hotmail.com
The Netherlands	www.vmbn.nl
	www.instituutvoormindfulness.nl
	www.fritskoster.nl
	www.ingridvandenhout.nl
	www.stillmotion-osteopathie.nl,
	www.aandachttrainingnijmegen.nl
	www.livingmindfulness.nl
	www.presentmind.nl
	http://aandachtvoordekern.nl
New Zealand	www.mentalhealth.org.nz/home/our-work
	/category/mindfulness
	www.wholistichealthworks.co.nz
	www.mindfulpsychology.co.nz
Northern Ireland	www.kridyom.uk
Norway	www.institute-for-mindfulness.org/mbsr/Find
	-an-MBSR-teacher-near-you
	www.nfon.no
	www.ntnu.edu/studies/mbsr-mbct-teacher-training
	www.mindfulness-laerere.no
Peru	www.concienciaplenaperu.com
Poland	www.institute-for-mindfulness.org/mbsr/Find-an
	-MBSR-teacher-near-you
	www.polski-instytut-mindfulness.pl
Slovakia	andrej.jelenik@gmail.com
Slovenia	www.dr-gross-online.info
South Africa	www.mindfulness.org.za
Spain	www.mbsr-instructores.org/miembros
	nirakara.org/mbsr

Sweden	www.mindfulnesscenter.se
	www.cfms.se
Switzerland	www.mbsr-verband.ch
	www.institute-for-mindfulness.org/mbsr/Find-an
	-MBSR-teacher-near-you
	www.centerformindfulness.ch
Taiwan	www.mindfulness.org.tw
	www.mindfulnesscenter.tw
	www.mbha.org.tw
Turkey	http://zumraatalay.com
	yardimci.beril@gmail.com
United Kingdom	www.institute-for-mindfulness.org/mbsr
	/Find-an-MBSR-teacher-near-you
	www.mindfulnessteachersuk.org.uk
	www.bangor.ac.uk/mindfulness

Index

The Institute for Mindfulness-Based Approaches

Founded by Linda Lehrhaupt, PhD, in 2001, the Institute for Mindfulness-Based Approaches is the oldest training institute of its kind on the European continent. Since its founding, it has grown to be one of the largest training institutes in mindfulness-based approaches in Europe. More than twelve hundred professionals alone have participated in its eighteen-month-long MBSR teacher-training program. Graduates of that and other programs it offers now teach in a wide variety of clinical, mental health, private practice, therapeutic, educational, rehabilitative, and social institutional settings.

At present, the IMA offers teacher-training programs in Mindfulness-Based Stress Reduction, Mindfulness-Based Cognitive Therapy, and Mindfulness-Based Compassionate Living in eight European countries. In Norway it offers an MBSR-MBCT teacher training course in cooperation with the National University of Science and Technology. The faculty of the IMA are among the most experienced in Europe. A number of the institute's faculty members are currently conducting research in various settings as well as publishing in their respective fields.

The IMA has also developed innovative continuing education programs for teachers of mindfulness-based approaches. These programs include mentoring for MBSR, MBCT, and MBCL (Mindfulness-Based Compassionate Living) teachers, as well as mindfulness meditation guidance for professionals working with mindfulness-based interventions. IMA faculty and guest teachers offer retreats in mindfulness meditation to support the personal practice of teachers and participants in their training programs.

The IMA is committed to fostering high-quality teacher training and strongly aligns itself with the training standards and ethical policy statement of the German MBSR-MBCT National Teachers Association, to the guidelines of the UK Mindfulness Teachers Network, as well as guideliness published on the website of the Center for Mindfulness in Medicine, Health Care, and Society. Dr. Lehrhaupt, the executive director of the IMA, serves on international committees to support the integrity of course standards and teacher competency in MBSR and MBCT.

www.institute-for-mindfulness.org (in English)
www.institut-fuer-achtsamkeit.de (in German)

The Ruhr Mindfulness Institute

The Ruhr Mindfulness Institute, a training institute for mindfulness-based approaches, was established in 2016 by Petra and Jörg Meibert and Prof. Dr. Johannes Michalak. Based on their long experience as mindfulness teachers, researchers, therapists, and MBSR-MBCT teacher trainers, the founders are committed to the highest standards of the training of teachers and the dissemination of mindfulness-based methods. They offer personal support during the training, qualified teachers with deep roots in the practice of mindfulness, and a scientific foundation. The institute collaborates with well-known cooperation partners.

The institute offers teacher training programs in MBSR, MBCT, and MBPM (Mindfulness-Based Pain Management — Breathworks Method). It also offers continuing education programs for MBSR and MBCT teachers as well as one-year mindfulness trainings for persons in therapeutic and educational professions, and eight-week courses in MBSR and MBCT.

www.achtsamkeitsinstitut-ruhr.de (in German)

About the Authors

Linda Lehrhaupt, PhD, is the founder and executive director of the Institute for Mindfulness-Based Approaches and one of Europe's most senior MBSR teachers. With almost thirty-five years of experience as a teacher and supervisor in mindfulness-based approaches, she has a rich background in their integration in education, health care, and personal development. She began teaching MBSR in 1993 and is certified to teach it by the Center for Mindfulness in Medicine, Health Care, and Society at the University of Massachusetts Medical School. She holds a degree in education and a PhD in performance studies, with a specialty in religious ritual and traditions. She is a founding member of the German National MBSR-MBCT Teachers Association and the European Network of Associations of Mindfulness-Based Approaches (EAMBA).

Dr. Lehrhaupt has been practicing Zen meditation since 1979 and is a teacher in the White Plum Lineage founded by Taizan Maezumi, Roshi. She received Dharma Transmission from Al Fusho Rapaport, Sensei, founder of Open Mind Zen, and also studied Zen for many years with Dennis Genpo Merzel, Roshi, and Nico Tydeman, Sensei. She is the guiding teacher for Zen Heart Sangha, an inter-European group of Zen practitioners, and has been leading retreats in Zen and in mindfulness meditation for many years.

In 1976 she fell in love with tai chi and qigong and went on to train with some of the leading representatives of the first generation of Asian teachers in the West. For over twenty years, beginning in 1982, she directed innovative teacher-training programs in tai chi and meditative movement, and she also developed Europe's first teacher-training program in qigong and women's health.

Dr. Lehrhaupt is the creator of the podcast series *Mindfulness-Based Teacher Project*, providing inspiration, support, and know-how to teachers of mindfulness-based approaches (www.mindfulness-based-teacher -project.org).

She is the author of *Riding the Waves of Life: Mindfulness and Inner Balance* (in German, 2012) and *Tai Chi as a Path of Wisdom* (in English, 2001); and she is coauthor of *MBSR: Reducing Stress through Mindfulness* (in German, 2010).

Dr. Lehrhaupt, who is American, has been living with her family in Germany since 1983. She also spends part of every year in the United States.

Contact: LindaLehrhaupt@aol.com
info@institute-for-mindfulness.org
www.institute-for-mindfulness.org
www.institut-fuer-achtsamkeit.de

Petra Meibert, Dipl. Psych., is a psychologist and one of Germany's leading experts on MBSR, MBCT (Mindfulness-Based Cognitive Therapy), and the applications of mindfulness in medicine and psychotherapy. She is cofounder and codirector of the Achtsamkeitsinstitut Ruhr, a German institute for mindfulness-based interventions, where she is involved in the MBSR and MBCT teacher-training programs. She completed her training as an MBSR teacher at the Institute for Mindfulness-Based Approaches and pursued further education and supervision at the Center for Mindfulness in Medicine, Health Care, and Society at the University of Massachusetts Medical School. Since 2005, she has had teaching experience both in Germany and internationally, especially in MBSR and MBCT teacher-training programs.

Since 1990 she has been integrating humanistic body-centered psychotherapeutic methods in her work with clients. She began teaching MBSR in 2003 and, shortly thereafter, MBCT. She has also been vice president of the board of the German National Association for MBSR and MBCT Teachers since 2005 and is involved in the development of the European Network of Associations of Mindfulness-Based Approaches (EAMBA).

She has participated in MBCT research projects at Ruhr University, Bochum, Germany, in relation to preventing the relapse of depression, and she worked at the University of Zurich, Switzerland, in a research project on the theme of trust, where she developed a questionnaire for the assessment of basic trust.

Petra Meibert studied Buddhist psychology and philosophy for several years with the Tibetan Buddhist teacher Tarab Tulku Rinpoche and has practiced mindfulness meditation, Vipassana, and Dzogchen since 1988.

She is the author of a German book on MBCT, *Finding a Way to Free Yourself from Rumination: Mindfulness Training for People Suffering from Depression, Anxiety and Negative Inner Monologues* (Kösel, 2014); and *Mindfulness-Based Therapy and Stress Reduction MBCT/MBSR: Ways in Psychotherapy* (Reinhardt Verlag, 2016). She is coauthor (with Ulrike Anderessen-Reuster and Sabine Meck) of *Psychotherapy and Buddhist Mind Training* (in German; Schattauer, 2013). She has also written articles about MBSR, MBCT, and mindfulness in various books and scientific journals, including the *Journal of Nervous and Mental Disease*.

Contact: j.p.meibert@t-online.de
or see
www.achtsamkeitsinstitut-ruhr.de.